P9-BYU-666

CHILD AND ADULT CARE FOOD PROGRAM

ALIGNING DIETARY GUIDANCE FOR ALL

Committee to Review Child and Adult Care Food Program
Meal Requirements

Food and Nutrition Board

Suzanne P. Murphy, Ann L. Yaktine,
Carol West Suitor, and Sheila Moats, *Editors*

INSTITUTE OF MEDICINE
OF THE NATIONAL ACADEMIES

THE NATIONAL ACADEMIES PRESS
Washington, D.C.
www.nap.edu

THE NATIONAL ACADEMIES PRESS   500 Fifth Street, N.W.   Washington, DC 20001

NOTICE: The project that is the subject of this report was approved by the Governing Board of the National Research Council, whose members are drawn from the councils of the National Academy of Sciences, the National Academy of Engineering, and the Institute of Medicine. The members of the committee responsible for the report were chosen for their special competences and with regard for appropriate balance.

This study was supported by Contract No. AG-3198-C-08-0001 between the National Academy of Sciences and the U.S. Department of Agriculture. Any opinions, findings, conclusions, or recommendations expressed in this publication are those of the author(s) and do not necessarily reflect the view of the organizations or agencies that provided support for this project.

International Standard Book Number-13:   978-0-309-15845-9
International Standard Book Number-10:   0-309-15845-1

Additional copies of this report are available from the National Academies Press, 500 Fifth Street, N.W., Lockbox 285, Washington, DC 20055; (800) 624-6242 or (202) 334-3313 (in the Washington metropolitan area); Internet, http://www.nap.edu.

For more information about the Institute of Medicine, visit the IOM home page at: **www.iom.edu.**

The serpent has been a symbol of long life, healing, and knowledge among almost all cultures and religions since the beginning of recorded history. The serpent adopted as a logotype by the Institute of Medicine is a relief carving from ancient Greece, now held by the Staatliche Museen in Berlin.

Suggested citation: IOM (Institute of Medicine). 2011. *Child and Adult Care Food Program: Aligning Dietary Guidance for All.* Washington, DC: The National Academies Press.

"Knowing is not enough; we must apply. Willing is not enough; we must do."

—Goethe

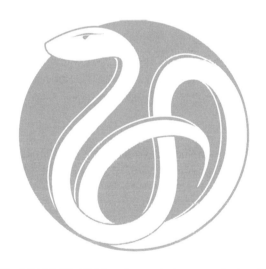

INSTITUTE OF MEDICINE
OF THE NATIONAL ACADEMIES

Advising the Nation. Improving Health.

THE NATIONAL ACADEMIES
Advisers to the Nation on Science, Engineering, and Medicine

The **National Academy of Sciences** is a private, nonprofit, self-perpetuating society of distinguished scholars engaged in scientific and engineering research, dedicated to the furtherance of science and technology and to their use for the general welfare. Upon the authority of the charter granted to it by the Congress in 1863, the Academy has a mandate that requires it to advise the federal government on scientific and technical matters. Dr. Ralph J. Cicerone is president of the National Academy of Sciences.

The **National Academy of Engineering** was established in 1964, under the charter of the National Academy of Sciences, as a parallel organization of outstanding engineers. It is autonomous in its administration and in the selection of its members, sharing with the National Academy of Sciences the responsibility for advising the federal government. The National Academy of Engineering also sponsors engineering programs aimed at meeting national needs, encourages education and research, and recognizes the superior achievements of engineers. Dr. Charles M. Vest is president of the National Academy of Engineering.

The **Institute of Medicine** was established in 1970 by the National Academy of Sciences to secure the services of eminent members of appropriate professions in the examination of policy matters pertaining to the health of the public. The Institute acts under the responsibility given to the National Academy of Sciences by its congressional charter to be an adviser to the federal government and, upon its own initiative, to identify issues of medical care, research, and education. Dr. Harvey V. Fineberg is president of the Institute of Medicine.

The **National Research Council** was organized by the National Academy of Sciences in 1916 to associate the broad community of science and technology with the Academy's purposes of furthering knowledge and advising the federal government. Functioning in accordance with general policies determined by the Academy, the Council has become the principal operating agency of both the National Academy of Sciences and the National Academy of Engineering in providing services to the government, the public, and the scientific and engineering communities. The Council is administered jointly by both Academies and the Institute of Medicine. Dr. Ralph J. Cicerone and Dr. Charles M. Vest are chair and vice chair, respectively, of the National Research Council.

www.national-academies.org

Reviewers

This report has been reviewed in draft form by individuals chosen for their diverse perspectives and technical expertise, in accordance with procedures approved by the National Research Council's Report Review Committee. The purpose of this independent review is to provide candid and critical comments that will assist the institution in making its published report as sound as possible and to ensure that the report meets institutional standards for objectivity, evidence, and responsiveness to the study charge. The review comments and draft manuscript remain confidential to protect the integrity of the deliberative process. We wish to thank the following individuals for their review of this report:

Denise M. Brown, Department of Nutrition and Food Systems, The University of Southern Mississippi, Hattiesburg

Jean Charles-Azure, Indian Health Service, Rockville, MD

Barbara L. Devaney, Mathematica Policy Research, Inc., Princeton, NJ

Craig Gundersen, Department of Agriculture and Consumer Education, University of Illinois, Urbana

James O. Hill, Center for Human Nutrition, Colorado Clinical Nutrition Research Unit, Denver

Nancy F. Krebs, Department of Pediatrics, Section of Nutrition, University of Colorado, Denver

Joanne R. Lupton, Department of Nutrition and Food Science, Texas A&M University, College Station

Although the reviewers listed above have provided many constructive comments and suggestions, they were not asked to endorse the conclusions or recommendations nor did they see the final draft of the report before its release. The review of this report was overseen by **Eileen Kennedy,** Friedman School of Nutrition Science and Policy, Tufts University, and **Jeanne Brooks-Gunn,** Teachers College and College of Physicians and Surgeons, Columbia University. Appointed by the National Research Council and Institute of Medicine, they were responsible for making certain that an independent examination of this report was carried out in accordance with institutional procedures and that all review comments were carefully considered. Responsibility for the final content of this report rests entirely with the authoring committee and the institution.

Preface

The Child and Adult Care Food Program (CACFP) is a U.S. Department of Agriculture (USDA) food program that is not well-known to either the general public or nutrition professionals. I must admit that I knew little about this program before the Committee to Review CACFP Meal Requirements began its work. I did not know that CACFP

- Serves almost 3 million children and adults,
- Has participants ranging in age from small infants to elderly adults, and
- Can provide over half of the day's calories for some participants through two meals and a snack, or two snacks and a meal.

Over the past year, as the committee carried out its tasks, my knowledge and appreciation for CACFP have grown enormously. Several members of the committee, including me, had served as members of the authoring committees for two other recent reviews of USDA's food programs: Special Supplemental Nutrition Program for Women, Infants, and Children (WIC) and the National School Lunch and Breakfast Programs. However, we still had much to understand about the uniqueness of CACFP. In this process, we were guided and informed by the expertise of committee members with many years of experience with the program. The resulting report was truly a team effort by experts from many disciplines: nutrition, epidemiology, statistics, economics, and food program implementation. I think I speak for the whole committee in saying it has been a very rewarding experience to participate in the review of the CACFP meal requirements. We hope that the resulting recommendations will help to make this excellent food program even better. Furthermore, given the broad scope of CACFP, these recommendations should be applicable across all age groups, and thus effectively align dietary guidance for all Americans.

The committee could not have done its work without the tireless efforts of the Institute of Medicine study team. The Study Director, Ann Yaktine, kept us focused and on time, and contributed substantially to the writing effort. She was assisted by an able team, including Sheila Moats, Associate Program Officer, who assisted with food pattern analysis; Julia Hoglund, Research Associate, who assisted with the cost analysis and research support; and Heather Breiner, Program Associate, who managed program logistics. Linda Meyers, the Director of the Food and Nutrition Board, provided us with wise advice at crucial points in our deliberations. Last, but certainly not least, Carol Suitor joined us as a consulting editor during the writing phase and made extensive contributions to the final report. I am grateful to all of them.

Other people made important contributions to the many analyses that were necessary for the report. Todd Campbell from Iowa State University developed the software that was used to determine the costs and helped with assigning codes to foods for the purpose of nutrient analyses, and Janice Maras from Northeastern University assisted with the menu analyses. In addition, we held an open session at our second meeting, and we heard from both the CACFP program administrators at the Food and Nutrition Service at USDA and from others with expertise relevant to the committee's task. Our thanks go to all who contributed to our deliberations.

Finally, as chair, I would like to express my sincere appreciation to the committee members for their commitment to making the report scientifically accurate as well as realistic and practical. The committee added this volunteer effort to their full-time jobs, and that often required working nights and weekends. I thank them for their time and many contributions. It was a pleasure working with each of them.

Suzanne P. Murphy, *Chair*
Committee to Review Child and Adult Care
Food Program Meal Requirements

Contents

*Appendixes D through M are not printed in this book but can be found on the CD at the back of the book or online at http://www.nap.edu.

Summary

The Child and Adult Care Food Program (CACFP) has the broadest scope of any of the U.S. Department of Agriculture (USDA) food programs. It supports the nutrition and health of our nation's most vulnerable populations—infants and children (especially those in low-income households) and adults who require daily supervision or assistance. Many of these participants rely on CACFP for the majority of their food intake, so the quality of the foods provided has the potential to substantially improve the overall adequacy and healthfulness of their diets. Furthermore, the availability of affordable care that includes meals and snacks of high nutritional quality provides an invaluable form of support for parents, guardians, or caregivers who need to be employed. CACFP currently serves approximately 3.3 million children and 114,000 adults across the United States. Yet, in spite of the importance of this program to millions of American families, the key role of CACFP in the food assistance spectrum is under-appreciated by both nutrition professionals and the public. To ensure that the meals and snacks provided by this crucial food program are of the highest quality possible, the USDA asked the Institute of Medicine (IOM) to review and recommend improvements, as necessary, to the Meal Requirements for CACFP.

Over the past decade, the federal government has sought the advice of the IOM to improve the nutrition and health opportunities for millions of Americans across a range of age, gender, and economic groups. In response, reports from the IOM have issued recommendations for

1

- Improved food packages provided through the Supplemental Nutrition Program for Women, Infants, and Children (WIC),
- Nutrition standards for competitive foods offered or sold in the school setting, and
- Revised Meal Requirements for the National School Lunch Program and the School Breakfast Program.

These recommendations are grounded in the sound nutritional guidance and nutrient standards of the current *Dietary Guidelines for Americans* and the Dietary Reference Intakes (DRIs). This study of CACFP is a follow-up of the study to recommend revised standards and requirements for school meals. Like WIC and the school meal programs, CACFP is a nutrition assistance program that is administered by the Food and Nutrition Service (FNS) of USDA. CACFP serves infants, preschool children, and children younger than 12 years in child care centers and homes, older children in at-risk afterschool programs and emergency shelters; and disabled and older adults in adult day care centers. CACFP is also broad in the types of meals provided, which may include breakfast, lunch, supper, and snacks. Finally, the settings for CACFP meals are diverse, ranging from small family day care homes to large day care centers and schools.

TASK AND APPROACH

USDA requested that the IOM convene a panel of experts to undertake a study to review and recommend revisions to the CACFP Meal Requirements. The major objective was to develop practical recommendations that would bring CACFP meals and snacks into alignment with current dietary guidance. Specifically, the committee was asked to

- Review and assess the nutritional needs of the target populations based on the *Dietary Guidelines for Americans* and the DRIs, and
- Use that review as a basis for recommended revisions to the Meal Requirements for CACFP.

As part of its task, the committee was asked to consider certain critical issues identified by the FNS. The committee's goal was to develop well-conceived, practical, and economical recommendations that reflect current nutritional science; to omit foods of low nutritional value; and to enhance the ability of the program to effectively meet the nutritional needs of the children and adults served.

Considering the broad scope of CACFP, the committee took a broad view of its assignment by developing Meal Requirements that could be used for specific meals and across a full day, that covered all age groups from infants through older adults, and that could be implemented both by providers in family homes and by those in large centers. The recommended Meal Requirements that are described in this report provide a framework that can be extended beyond CACFP and used to design and implement other food and nutrition recommendations in a variety of settings and programs as the need arises.

To address its task, the committee formulated a strategy that included the review of published literature and other available evidence, consideration of information from public workshop presentations, analyses of relevant data, and deliberations on topics relevant to its charge. Prior to proposing revisions to the CACFP Meal Requirements, the committee developed criteria to guide its deliberations. Box S-1 presents the five criteria that guided the decision-making process used to generate the committee's recommendations.

BOX S-1
CACFP Criteria

Criterion 1. The Meal Requirements will be consistent with current dietary guidance and nutrition recommendations to promote health with the ultimate goal of improving participants' diets by reducing the prevalence of inadequate and excessive intakes of food, nutrients, and calories.

  a. For infants and children younger than 2 years of age, the Meal Requirements will contribute to an overall diet that is consistent with established dietary recommendations for this age group and encourage and support breastfeeding for infants.
  b. For participating adults and children ages 2 years and older, the Meal Requirements will be consistent with the *Dietary Guidelines for Americans* and the Dietary Reference Intakes.

Criterion 2. The Meal Requirements will provide the basis for menus that are practical to plan, purchase, prepare, and serve in different settings.

Criterion 3. The Meal Requirements will provide the basis for menus that incorporate healthful foods and beverages and are appealing to diverse age ranges and cultural backgrounds.

Criterion 4. The Meal Requirements will facilitate the planning of menus that are compatible with the capabilities and resources for the variety of program providers.

Criterion 5. The Meal Requirements will allow the planning of menus that are sensitive to considerations of cost.

TABLE S-1 Recommended Age Groups for CACFP Meal Patterns

Age Group	Age Range[a]
Infants	0–5 months
	6–11 months
Children	1 year
	2–4 years
	5–13 years[b]
	14–18 years[b]
Adults	19 years and older

[a]Age ranges are inclusive; e.g., ages 0–5 months includes ages 0 *through* 5 months.

[b]The committee recognizes that children older than 12 years ordinarily are eligible only for the at-risk afterschool program, but migrant children are eligible through age 15 years, and youths in shelters are eligible to age 18 years.

Process to Develop Recommendations

An iterative process was used to develop recommendations for revised CACFP Meal Requirements. The first step was to set key parameters, including age groups and total daily calorie requirements. Then the current intakes of individuals in these age groups were evaluated by comparison to standards for food groups and nutrient intakes. This was done to identify food and nutrient intakes of concern. Next, nutrient and food group intake targets for CACFP were developed, taking into account the identified nutritional needs of the CACFP population. Finally, meal patterns and food specifications were developed to be used as the basis of the recommended Meal Requirements for CACFP. This last step was repeated until the new Meal Requirements aligned with the *Dietary Guidelines for Americans* and the DRIs.

As a part of this process, the committee considered the five criteria in Box S-1 and the unique aspects of the program. Importantly, the committee gave consideration to the practicality and cost of implementing revisions to the program in the different types of settings in which CACFP operates.

Age Groups

The age groups for which patterns are recommended are similar to those currently used by CACFP, although some changes have been made for the younger children to correspond to recent dietary guidance. See Table S-1 for the recommended age groups.

RECOMMENDATIONS

As structured by the committee, the recommended Meal Requirements encompass two distinct elements: meal patterns and food specifications.

The Meal Requirements serve to (1) provide patterns and specifications for menus consistent with the *Dietary Guidelines* and nutrient targets and (2) allow the identification of meals that qualify for reimbursement. Recommendations for Meal Requirements, implementation strategies, and evaluation and research are addressed below.

Recommendations for Revised Meal Requirements: Meal Patterns and Food Specifications

In order to bring the Meal Requirements into alignment with the best available dietary guidance and to improve consistency with the requirements of other FNS programs, the committee recommends that the FNS of USDA take the following steps:

Meal Requirement Recommendation 1: **USDA should adopt the recommended Meal Requirements for healthy infants up to 1 year of age.** Key elements of this recommendation are the provision of only breast milk or formula for infants under 6 months of age; the gradual introduction of baby meats, cereals, fruits, and vegetables beginning at age 6 months; and the omission of fruit juice of any type before the age of 1 year. Tables 7-1 and 7-8 in Chapter 7 provide the detailed specifications for the infant meal patterns.

Meal Requirement Recommendation 2: **For all children age 1 year and older and for adults, USDA should adopt Meal Requirements that increase the variety of fruits and vegetables, increase the proportion of whole grains, and decrease the content of solid fats, added sugars, *trans* fats, and sodium.** The recommended Meal Requirements continue to contain valuable features of the current meal requirements, such as focusing on food groups, specifying minimum amounts of foods to be provided at meals and snacks, and not allowing foods such as soft drinks, fruit drinks, and candy to be included in reimbursable meals. Three types of meal patterns continue to be defined: breakfast, lunch and supper, and snacks. The major food groups in the meal patterns are also similar to those currently used: fruits and vegetables, grains/bread, meat/meat alternates, and milk (but fruits and vegetables are now separated in the pattern specifications). Although the foods contained in these groups continue to be like the MyPyramid food groups and cheese and yogurt still may be used as meat alternates, there is an emphasis on lean or low fat choices. The new recommended food specifications place limitations on a larger number of foods within each food group.

As with the current meal patterns, differences in energy and nutrient needs across the age groups for children and adults are considered by adjusting the portion sizes within the food groups. The amount of food in the meal patterns increases across the four younger age groups (age 1 year, 2–4 years, 5–13 years, and 14–18 years), and then decreases for adults to

BOX S-2
Recommended Daily Meal Patterns for
Breakfast, Lunch/Supper, and Snacks: Number
of Servings and Range of Serving Sizes[a]

Food Group	Serving Number	Range of Serving Size
Breakfast		
Fruit or non-starchy vegetable	1	¼ to ½ cup
Grains/breads	1	½ to 3 ounce equivalent
Lean meat/meat alternate	1	½ to 2 ounce equivalent (3 times weekly)
Milk	1	½ to 1 cup
Lunch/Supper		
Fruit	1	¼ to ½ cup
Vegetable	2	⅛ to ½ cup
Grains/breads	1	½ to 2-½ ounce equivalent
Lean meat/meat alternate	1	½ to 2-½ ounce equivalent
Milk	1	½ to 1 cup
Snacks		
(Choose 2 Food Groups per Snack)		
Fruit	2 per week	½ to 1 cup
Vegetable	2 per week	⅛ to 1 cup
Grains/breads	2 per week	½ to 2 ounce equivalent
Lean meat/meat alternate	2 per week	½ to 1 ounce equivalent
Milk	2 per week	½ cup

[a]Serving sizes vary by age group

approximately the same level as for children 5–13 years of age. In addition, for several of the food groups, the amounts of food within the group are similar to those specified for the current meal patterns. Box S-2 shows the basic format of the meal patterns and the ranges of portion sizes across age groups. Tables 7-2 through 7-8 provide more details on these patterns.

However, within this framework for meal patterns and food specifications, several new elements are being recommended, as follows:

a.   One fruit and two different vegetables are to be served at each lunch and supper meal. Over the course of a 5-day week, different types of vegetables are to be served at each lunch and supper,

   as follows: dark green vegetables at least twice per week, orange
   vegetables at least twice per week, legumes at least once per week,
   starchy vegetables no more than twice per week, and other vegetables at least three times per week.
   b. Fruit rather than fruit juice is to be served at most meals; juice must
       be unsweetened 100 percent juice and is allowed only once per day
       in a serving size tailored to the age group's needs.
   c. At least half of the grains/breads served in meals and snacks must
       be whole grain-rich, meeting the definition given in the table of
       proposed food specifications (Table 7-8). Other grain/bread must
       be enriched. Providers are encouraged to gradually increase the
       proportion of grain foods that are whole grain-rich to well above
       half of the grain foods and to include 100 percent whole grain
       foods often.
   d. Each morning and afternoon snack will provide two different food
       components in a serving size tailored to the age group's needs; over
       the course of a 5-day week, the food components provided will
       include two servings of fruit, one serving of an orange vegetable,
       one serving of a non-starchy vegetable, two servings of grain/bread,
       two servings of lean meat or meat alternate, and two servings of
       low-fat or nonfat milk.
   e. The amounts of solid fats, added sugars, *trans* fats, and sodium are
       to be limited in all meals and snacks. For example, milk and yogurt
       must be low fat or nonfat for those ages 2 years or older (whole
       milk for 1-year-old children), meats must be lean, fruits and juices
       must be free of added sugars, foods with nutritional labels must
       be labeled as containing zero grams of *trans* fat, and foods high in
       added sugars and/or sodium are to be served infrequently, if at all.
   f. Meat or meat alternates are to be served at breakfast three times a
       week. Table 7-8, in Chapter 7 gives the specifications for lean meat
       and low-fat cooking methods.

   Although the major food groups in each meal are served every day,
specific selections within the food groups vary across the days of the week,
as do the snack selections. As a result, the committee notes that weekly
menu planning would help providers achieve the specified variety and adopt
efficient new shopping patterns and ways to control costs.
   As shown in Table S-2, the recommended Meal Requirements differ
in many important ways from those in the current regulations. They are
much more consistent with current dietary guidance and nutrition recommendations to promote health. The committee's recommendations create a
comprehensive system of requirements focusing control on the specific food

TABLE S-2 Comparison of Current Requirements with Recommended Meal Requirements and Specifications

Eating Occasion	Current Requirements	Recommended Requirements and Specifications
All	Must meet daily pattern	Must meet daily and weekly patterns to provide more flexibility and better alignment with the *Dietary Guidelines*
Breakfast	3 meal components	4 or 5 meal components
Lunch or supper	4 meal components	5 meal components
Snack	Any 2 of 4 components	Variety specified for the week Choice between 2 small snacks or 1 enhanced snack
Meal Component		
Fruit	Fruits and vegetables are combined as a category	Fruits are a separate category, and servings are increased; juice is not provided for infants and is limited for children; fruits containing added sugars are limited
Vegetable		Vegetables are a separate category from fruit, and servings are increased; must provide variety including dark green leafy, bright yellow/orange, legumes; sodium content is limited; starchy vegetables are limited
Grain	Enriched or whole grain, proportions not specified	At least half must be whole grain-rich; additional whole grains are encouraged; grain products high in solid fats and added sugars are limited to control calories and saturated fat; high-sodium grain products are also limited
Meat/alternate	None at breakfast No restrictions on high-fat, highly processed meats	Included in weekly breakfast pattern Some types are limited to help control calories, solid fat, and sodium

TABLE S-2 Continued

Eating Occasion	Current Requirements	Recommended Requirements and Specifications
Milk	Any type of fluid milk	Must be nonfat or low-fat (1% fat) for children over 2 years of age and adults, whole milk for 1-year-old children Flavored milk must be nonfat and is allowed only for at-risk and afterschool programs and adult programs A limited amount of nonfat or low-fat yogurt is allowed as a milk substitute for children over 2 years of age and adults, if not used as a meat substitute
Food Component		
Energy	No requirement	Calories are controlled by limiting foods high in solid fats and added sugars
Micronutrients	No standard specified by regulation	Meal patterns are designed to achieve, for protein and most micronutrients, DRI targets consistent with a low prevalence of inadequacy
Fats	No restriction on type of amount	Label must state zero *trans* fat (if applicable); food specifications limit highly processed and high fat meats and foods; moderate use of healthy fats is encouraged
Sodium	No restriction	No salt at the table Recommendations to choose commercial foods low in sodium and to prepare foods with less salt

NOTE: DRI = Dietary Reference Intake.

groups and variety of key subgroups offered for all meals and snacks and on the nutrition quality of all foods served through food specifications.

By convening a panel of expert CACFP sponsors, providers, state administrators, and CACFP associations (see Appendix M), and trainers, it is possible that USDA could identify a process for phasing in some of the more complex new elements with the goal of supporting the recommended Meal Requirements.

Meal Requirement Recommendation 3: **USDA should give CACFP providers the option of serving one enhanced snack in the afternoon in place of a smaller snack in both the morning and the afternoon.** The enhanced snack option (shown in Table 7-6) would be particularly appropriate for at-risk children in afterschool programs and for older adults because their access to nutritious foods may be limited at home. The enhanced snack would have the same requirements as two of the smaller snacks. Providers would specify in advance which snack option they were choosing, and would serve the same type of snack to all participants in their care.

Recommendations for Implementation Strategies

In order to bring the Meal Requirements into alignment with the best available guidance and improve their consistency with the nutritional requirements of other programs of the FNS, the committee makes the following recommendations.

Implementation Strategy Recommendation 1: **USDA, working together with state agencies and health and professional organizations, should provide extensive technical assistance to CACFP providers to implement the recommended Meal Requirements.** Key aspects of new technical assistance to providers include measures to continuously improve menu planning (including variety in vegetable servings and snack offerings across the week), purchasing, food preparation, and record keeping. Such assistance will be essential to enable providers to meet the Meal Requirements while controlling cost and maintaining quality. Many potential partners and resources are available that USDA could tap to assist with developing training materials and/or provide the training. Some of these are listed in Appendix M.

Implementation Strategy Recommendation 2: **USDA should work strategically with the CACFP administering state agencies, CACFP associations, and other stakeholders to reevaluate and streamline the system for monitoring and reimbursing CACFP meals and snacks.** The CACFP National Professional Association and the Child and Adult Care Food Program Sponsor's Association would be key partners. Several aspects of the existing monitoring and reimbursement processes will need to be revised to enable states to efficiently administer the CACFP program with the new recommended Meal Requirements in place. The procedures would be expected to (1) focus on meeting relevant *Dietary Guidelines* and (2) provide information for continuous quality improvement and for mentoring program operators to assist in performance improvement. Among the challenges will be the development of practical methods for states to monitor for compliance with weekly requirements and for minimizing providers' reporting requirements.

Recommendations for Program Evaluation and Research

While conducting this study, the committee encountered a considerable lack of up-to-date data relevant to CACFP, including participant characteristics, nutrient intake profiles, program costs, and certain program outcomes. The committee identified a need to improve data-gathering in all aspects of the program. In addition, a need was identified for ongoing evaluation of program standards and implementation efforts. Thus, the committee recommends that USDA take the following steps.

Program Evaluation Recommendation 1: **USDA, in collaboration with relevant agencies, should provide support for research to evaluate the impact of the Meal Requirements on participants' total and program-related dietary intake and consumption patterns, on the food and nutrient content of the meals and snacks served, on demand from eligible providers to participate in CACFP, and on program access by participants.** This evaluation would determine: (a) the food and nutrient content of meals and snacks as served, (b) participants' overall food and nutrient intakes as related to current dietary guidance, and (c) the number of providers and participants in the CACFP program.

Program Evaluation Recommendation 2: **USDA should take appropriate actions to establish the current baselines prior to implementation of the new Meal Requirements for comparison purposes.** Collection of a nationally representative baseline database of foods actually served is crucial. It will also be important to collect information on significant factors that might influence the impact of CACFP, including the number and types of meals served by age and setting, variations in state licensing requirements, and differences in the cost of living. Comparing CACFP child care to non-CACFP child care in the same geographic location could also contribute to fully understanding the impact of CACFP.

Program Evaluation Recommendation 3: **To the extent possible, USDA should take steps to ensure that the final rule for the new Meal Requirements is informed by the results of evaluation of program impact** (described in Recommendation 1 above). It will be critically important to evaluate the extent to which implementation of the revised Meal Requirements achieves the goal of promoting health and improving participants' diets by reducing the prevalence of inadequate and excessive intakes of foods, nutrients, and calories and contributing to an overall diet consistent with established dietary recommendations, including the *Dietary Guidelines for Americans*.

Research Recommendation 1: USDA, in collaboration with relevant agencies and foundations, should support research on topics related to the implementation of the Meal Requirements and to fill important gaps in knowledge of the role of CACFP in meeting the nutritional needs of program participants.

Research Recommendation 2: USDA should review and update, as appropriate, the CACFP Meal Requirements to maintain consistency with the *Dietary Guidelines* and other relevant science.

CONSISTENCY OF RECOMMENDATIONS WITH CRITERIA

The recommendations for Meal Requirements for CACFP and for implementing and monitoring them were evaluated for consistency with the committee's criteria, as summarized below. The committee worked to achieve an appropriate balance between competing aspects of the criteria, such as increased amounts of certain types of food, practicality, and cost.

Criterion 1: Consistency with Dietary Guidance

Recommendations for infants and children younger than 2 years of age reflect guidance from the American Academy of Pediatrics and result in feedings or meals that are in alignment with the DRIs. The Meal Requirements for those 2 years of age and older were designed to come as close as possible to *Dietary Guidelines* and to nutrient targets that were based on the DRIs while still being practical. Estimates of the nutrient content of the recommended sample menus indicated reasonable agreement with the nutrient targets, with the notable exception of sodium, vitamin E, and potassium. Review of the meal patterns and menus developed from the recommended Meal Requirements shows improved alignment with *Dietary Guidelines* (see Box S-3). The high nutrient quality of the meals contributes to the major role that CACFP plays in supporting the nutrition of those in day care and other CACFP settings.

Criterion 2: Practicality in Terms of
Planning, Purchasing, Preparing, and Serving Meals

The committee acknowledges that the recommended Meal Requirements are more complex than the current requirements, especially with regard to meal planning, even though adjustments were made to keep them as simple as possible. An increase in complexity is absolutely essential to achieve greater consistency with the *Dietary Guidelines*. For example, the

---

BOX S-3
Recommended Meal Requirements Improve
Alignment with the *Dietary Guidelines*

- Better control of calories
- More fruits and more vegetables
- A greater variety of vegetables
- More whole grain-rich foods, fewer refined grain foods
- Milk choices limited to nonfat and low fat; no flavored milk for younger children
- Increased emphasis on limiting foods high in solid fats and added sugars
- Minimized content of *trans* fat
- Stronger emphasis on gradual reduction of sodium

---

recommended meal pattern was revised to cover a 5 day week as well as a single day. This increase in complexity is one of the reasons for the recommendations related to technical assistance and monitoring. Reduced use of pre-prepared foods and increased in-house food preparation would be helpful in reducing sodium, solid fats, added sugars, and cost; technical assistance would help develop the skills needed.

Criterion 3: Appeal to Diverse Age Groups and Cultures

The meal patterns allow broad flexibility in planning menus. This means, for example, that those providers who serve preschool children can meet the pattern with a selection of foods that are suitable for their stage of development and that providers who serve the elderly can meet the pattern with an entirely different selection of foods if appropriate to the circumstances. The meal patterns developed by the committee are intended to allow for the inclusion of foods enjoyed by different cultures.

Criterion 4: Compatibility with the
Capabilities and Resources of Program Providers

The committee developed the standards for menu planning with the intent of making them adaptable to different provider venues: day care homes, centers, and other facilities such as Head Start. In the short term, program providers may face challenges in obtaining acceptable products, especially whole grain-rich foods and foods that are reduced in solid fats, added sugars, and sodium. This is a particular concern for day care settings with limited shopping options. Providers in all venues will need training and other types of support to plan menus that meet the recommended Meal Requirements and that are realistic for their situation.

Criterion 5: Sensitive to Cost

The recommended Meal Requirements increase overall food costs in CACFP mainly because of increased amounts and variety of fruits and vegetables for many age groups at lunch/supper and snacks, the addition of meat/meat alternates at breakfast (balanced only in part by reductions of meat/meat alternates at lunch for the younger children), and increases in the amount of whole grain-rich foods for some age groups. For example, using 2003–2004 prices, the combined cost of breakfast, lunch, and a regular snack is estimated to increase by $0.30, or 31 percent, for children 1 year of age, and by $0.56, or 44 percent, for children 2–4 years of age.

Non-food meal costs are expected to increase initially, to vary with the provider setting and with the extent to which the provider has already implemented changes similar to those recommended, and to be influenced substantially by the quality and extent of technical assistance provided. An increased need for training may persist but will be accompanied by improvements in food service and nutrition education, especially in larger centers.

The expected increase in costs will likely exceed the amount that can be absorbed by CACFP providers under current federal reimbursement levels. If the recommended Meal Requirements are fully implemented, continued participation by most providers will require an increase in reimbursement.

CONCLUSION

The new recommended Meal Requirements (meal patterns and food specification standards) will result in menus that are more closely aligned with the *Dietary Guidelines for Americans* and the DRIs than are the menus based on the current regulations. Notably, the recommended Meal Requirements may increase the consumption of fruits, vegetables, whole grain-rich foods, and lean meats, while decreasing the intake of solid fats, added sugars, and sodium. Initially, however, most providers will need considerable technical assistance in order to implement the recommended Meal Requirements without undue difficulty. With appropriate reimbursement and implementation strategies, the committee anticipates that providers' acceptance of the recommended changes in meals and snacks are achievable and that participation rates can be maintained or enhanced.

1

Introduction

The U.S. Department of Agriculture (USDA) Child and Adult Care Food Program (CACFP) is a federally sponsored program designed to provide healthy meals and snacks to children and adults receiving day care at participating family day care homes, traditional child care centers, at-risk afterschool care facilities, outside school hours care facilities, adult care facilities, and emergency shelters. Figure 1-1 shows the relative proportion of different facilities that participate in CACFP. Participating sites receive federal reimbursement for the meals and snacks they serve if the CACFP standards are met. In fiscal year 2010, the program served more than 3 million children and 114,000 functionally impaired adults and other adults over the age of 60 years. The total costs for the program in 2010 were approximately $2.2 billion (USDA/FNS, 2010, Tables 11, 15c, and 15d).

CACFP plays a critical role in improving day care for children and elderly or disabled adults. The benefits of CACFP include the following:

- Day care programs receive reimbursement for food served, which helps the programs to control their costs and offer more reasonable rates;
- As a result, care is more affordable for those who need it—in many cases enabling the child's or adult's primary care provider to work outside the home;
- CACFP regulations help ensure the nutritional quality and safety of the food served;

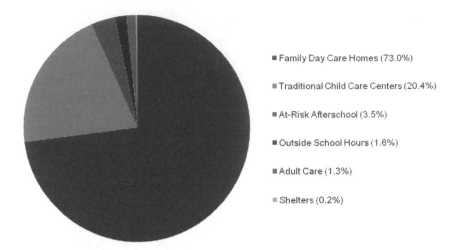

FIGURE 1 Percentage of various types of facilities participating in CACFP.
SOURCE: USDA/FNS, 2009.

- CACFP helps make afterschool programs more appealing to at-risk youth by offering nutritious snacks[1] in programs serving low-income areas (USDA/FNS, 2000); and
- Many CACFP participants also utilize other food programs; consistency in nutrition messages and nutritional benefits contribute to healthier outcomes for participants.

THE COMMITTEE'S TASK

Background

This study is the latest of a series of Institute of Medicine (IOM) studies that USDA has funded as a part of its multipronged effort to update regulations and guidance for several of its food programs. The updates are needed to bring the programs into better alignment with *Dietary Guidelines for Americans* (DGAs) (HHS/USDA, 2005) and with the nutrient reference standards called Dietary Reference Intakes (DRIs). In August 2008, the Food and Nutrition Service (FNS) of USDA asked the IOM's Food and Nutrition Board to make recommendations for CACFP meal requirements. This study augments the work done by the IOM to provide recommendations to revise the Nutrition Standards and Meal Requirements for the National School Lunch Program (NSLP) and the School Breakfast Program

---

[1]Suppers also may be offered now in 14 states.

(SBP), as covered in the report *School Meals: Building Blocks for Healthy Children* (IOM, 2010).

Statement of Task

Specifically, USDA requested that the IOM convene a panel of experts to

- Review and assess the nutritional needs of the target populations based on the *Dietary Guidelines for Americans* and the Dietary Reference Intakes, and
- Use that review as a basis for recommended revisions to the meal requirements for the Child and Adult Care Food Programs.

As part of its task, the committee was asked to consider certain critical issues identified by the FNS of USDA (Appendix D). The committee's goal was to develop well-conceived, practical, and economical recommendations that reflect current nutritional science; to increase the content of key food groups in the meals provided, as appropriate; and to allow the program to effectively meet the nutritional needs of the children and adults served.

Approach to the Task

To address its task, the committee reviewed published literature and other available evidence and drew information from public workshop presentations (see Appendix C). In addition, the committee contracted for nutrient and cost analyses of data based on the National Health and Nutrition Examination Survey (NHANES) 2004–2005 and data collected from CACFP programs (Food Research and Action Center, Washington, DC, contributed by G. Henchy, February 23, 2010). The committee formulated a strategy to address the scope of work, conducted analyses, and deliberated on issues relevant to its charge. To guide its deliberations and evaluate possible recommendations, the committee developed a set of criteria, presented in Chapter 6. The process and findings are described in detail in Chapter 7.

RATIONALE FOR REVISING THE MEAL REQUIREMENTS

The three major reasons for revising the meal requirements for CACFP are to

1. Improve alignment with current dietary guidance;
2. Achieve satisfactory consistency with standards and regulations of

three other USDA nutrition programs (the Supplemental Nutrition Program for Women, Infants, and Children [WIC], the NSLP, and the SBP) and with recommendations for competitive foods offered or sold in schools proposed in the report *Nutrition Standards for Foods in Schools* (IOM, 2007); and

3. Address the high prevalence of [childhood] obesity and other health concerns that result from limited access to nutritious foods.

These three topics are addressed on the following pages.

Changes in Dietary Guidance

The CACFP regulations were based in part on guidance in *Diet and Health* (NRC, 1989a) and on the 1989 *Recommended Dietary Allowances* (NRC, 1989b). Since the 1980s, many changes have been made in the three major sources of dietary guidance: (1) the *Dietary Guidelines for Americans*, source of federal nutrition policy; (2) the DRIs, intake recommendations that form the basis of U.S. dietary guidance; and (3) feeding recommendations from the American Academy of Pediatrics (AAP) for infants and children younger than 2 years of age.

Dietary Guidelines for Americans

Alignment with the *Dietary Guidelines* is essential because the guidelines form the basis of U.S. federal nutrition policy. In particular P.L. 101-445, Section 3 (7 U.S.C. 5341, the National Nutrition Monitoring and Related Research Act of 1990, Title III), directs the Secretaries of USDA and the Department of Health and Human Services (HHS) to issue jointly at least every 5 years a report entitled *Dietary Guidelines for Americans*. This law states that the DGA form the basis of federal food, nutrition education, and information programs. The most recent edition of the *Dietary Guidelines* was published in 2005 (HHS/USDA, 2005), and the release of the 2010 edition is expected in 2011. Compared with the 1985 *Dietary Guidelines* (HHS/USDA, 1985), which were in effect when CACFP regulations were established, the 2005 *Dietary Guidelines* are more quantitative and place stronger emphasis on the following:

- adequate calories within energy needs;
- controlling calorie intake to manage body weight;
- daily physical activity;
- increasing daily intake of fruits, vegetables, whole grains, and nonfat or low-fat milk and milk products;

- choosing fats wisely for good health;
- choosing carbohydrates wisely for good health;
- choosing and preparing foods with little salt;
- keeping alcohol intake moderate, if alcohol is consumed; and
- keeping food safe to eat.

Recommendations from the 2010 Dietary Guidelines Advisory Committee (USDA/HHS, 2010) are similar to the above but include even stronger emphasis on weight management, limiting intake of foods that are high in solid fats and added sugars, and reducing salt (sodium) intake. Further information about the 2005 Dietary Guidelines is available at http://www. cnpp.usda.gov/DietaryGuidelines.htm (accessed December 31, 2009). Detailed information about translating the *Dietary Guidelines* into meal patterns is provided by MyPyramid (HHS/USDA, 2005). Notably, both the *Dietary Guidelines* and MyPyramid apply to the general population ages 2 years and older but not to the younger children served by CACFP.

Dietary Reference Intakes

In 1994, the IOM developed a new paradigm for nutrient reference values that replaced the long established Recommended Dietary Allowances (RDAs) for the United States and the Recommended Nutrient Intakes (RNIs) for Canada. The new reference values, known as DRIs, differ from the RDAs and RNIs in several important ways. For example, the DRIs comprise a number of nutrient-based reference values, described in Chapter 3, that serve different purposes and are used in new ways. These reference values, along with descriptive text, are contained in six volumes published by the IOM between 1997 and 2005 (IOM, 1997, 1998, 2000, 2001, 2002/2005, 2005).

American Academy of Pediatrics

The American Academy of Pediatrics (AAP) Committee on Nutrition develops guidelines on the nutritional needs of infants, children, and adolescents. The AAP Committee works together with federal agencies including the HHS Food and Drug Administration, USDA, the HHS Centers for Disease Control and Prevention, the HHS National Institutes of Health, and the Canadian Paediatric Society to pursue advocacy opportunities that promote healthy dietary habits and provide technical assistance to facilitate relevant federal regulatory processes. The AAP Committee on Nutrition provides guidance on infant feeding, including breastfeeding, through its policy statements and its publication *Pediatric Nutrition Handbook* (AAP, 2009).

Consistency with Standards for WIC Food Packages and for Foods and Meals in Schools

Recent changes in several types of standards related to USDA nutrition assistance programs have been made or proposed to align the standards with current dietary guidance. In particular, new standards have been developed for WIC, and the IOM has proposed standards for competitive foods offered or sold in schools (IOM, 2007) and for the two major school meal programs: the NSLP and the SBP (IOM, 2010). One of the intended outcomes of new recommendations for CACFP meal requirements is to achieve consistent nutrition messages across programs.

Revised Regulations for WIC Food Packages

New WIC regulations have revised the WIC food packages to supply a set of foods that should help reduce both inadequate and excessive nutrient intake and contribute to a dietary pattern consistent with the current *Dietary Guidelines*. The regulations are based largely on recommendations made in the IOM report *WIC Food Packages: Time for a Change* (IOM, 2006). The revised packages allow more flexibility in the selection of certain types of food and include changes designed to support and promote the breastfeeding of infants.

Recommended Nutrition Standards for Foods in Schools

The report *Nutrition Standards for Foods in Schools: Leading the Way Toward Healthier Youth* (IOM, 2007) presents IOM recommendations, using a tiered approach, for nutrition standards for competitive foods offered or sold in schools. The standards were developed to encourage school-aged children and adolescents to consume foods and beverages that are healthful and to limit food components in competitive foods and beverages that are not healthful when consumed at levels that fall outside the current *Dietary Guidelines*. The proposed standards were developed for individual foods, not for meals. In addition, recommendations were made to limit the use of non-nutritive sweeteners and caffeine in foods offered in competition with school meal programs. Subsequent to the release of the IOM report, many school districts and several states have adopted new nutrition standards for competitive foods offered or sold in schools.

Recommended Requirements for School Meals

Currently, USDA is developing new meal requirements for the NSLP and SBP, using the IOM report *School Meals: Building Blocks for Healthy*

Children (IOM, 2010) as a major resource. The recommendations contained in *School Meals*, like those in the above-mentioned IOM reports relating to WIC and foods offered or sold in schools, focus on providing standards that are aligned with the current *Dietary Guidelines* and the DRIs, but in this case the focus is on complete meals.

Concern About Childhood Obesity

As discussed in Chapter 4, the prevalence of childhood obesity is much higher than it was when the current regulations for CACFP were adopted. The availability of foods and beverages at home, in a care center, or in any other location affects the overall quality of a child's diet and patterns of growth and weight gain. Thus, the type, nutritional quality, and amount of foods offered through CACFP are important factors that influence nutritional health.

Over the past several years, considerable research has been conducted to evaluate the nutritional effects of the consumption of foods that are low in nutrients but high in energy content (often called low-nutrient, energy-dense foods). Two studies (Drewnowski and Specter, 2004; Micch et al., 2006) indicate that the consumption of low-nutrient, energy-dense foods and irregular meal consumption patterns are contributing factors to the high prevalence of childhood obesity. Another study examined the types and amounts of beverages consumed by preschool children (O'Connor et al., 2006). This study, based on NHANES 1999–2002 data, found that the average milk consumption for preschool children was less than amounts recommended by the *Dietary Guidelines*, and that increased consumption of all beverages, including fruit juice and other sweetened drinks and soda, was associated with increased energy intake. Clearly, it was important for the committee to consider the nutrient and energy content of foods and beverages in developing its recommendations for meal requirements and food specifications for CACFP.

ORGANIZATION OF THE REPORT

The report is organized into 11 chapters. This chapter briefly introduced CACFP and provided a description of the committee's task and the rationale for the study. Chapter 2 describes CACFP in more detail and provides an overview of how CACFP contributes to the food and nutrition safety net that is provided by USDA's food assistance programs. Chapter 3 reviews and summarizes methods to examine food and nutrient intakes. Chapters 4 and 5 consider nutritional concerns for infants and children, and adults, respectively. Chapter 6 describes the process for developing recommendations for meal requirements, and Chapter 7 presents the recommendations for Meal Requirements. Chapter 8 contains an examination of cost implications and market effects relevant to CACFP meal requirements. Chapter 9 discusses implementation, and Chapter 10 compares the recommendations to the committee's working criteria. Chapter 11 presents recommendations for evaluation and future research. Additional material is provided in the appendixes.

REFERENCES

AAP (American Academy of Pediatrics). 2009. *Pediatric Nutrition Handbook*, 6th ed. Elk Grove Village, IL: AAP.

Drewnowski, A., and S. E. Specter. 2004. Poverty and obesity: The role of energy density and energy costs. *American Journal of Clinical Nutrition* 79(1):6–16.

HHS/USDA (U.S. Department of Health and Human Services/U.S. Department of Agriculture). 1985. *Nutrition and Your Health: Dietary Guidelines for Americans*, 2nd ed. Washington, DC: Government Printing Office. http://www.cnpp.usda.gov/Publications/DietaryGuidelines/1985/DG1985pub.pdf (accessed June 29, 2010).

HHS/USDA. 2005. *Dietary Guidelines for Americans*, 6th ed. Washington, DC: U.S. Government Printing Office. http://www.health.gov/DietaryGuidelines/dga2005/document/ (accessed July 23, 2008).

IOM (Institute of Medicine). 1997. *Dietary Reference Intakes for Calcium, Phosphorus, Magnesium, Vitamin D, and Fluoride*. Washington, DC: National Academy Press.

IOM. 1998. *Dietary Reference Intakes for Thiamin, Riboflavin, Niacin, Vitamin B_6, Folate, Vitamin B_{12}, Pantothenic Acid, Biotin, and Choline*. Washington, DC: National Academy Press.

IOM. 2000. *Dietary Reference Intakes for Vitamin C, Vitamin E, Selenium, and Carotenoids*. Washington, DC: National Academy Press.

IOM. 2001. *Dietary Reference Intakes for Vitamin A, Vitamin K, Arsenic, Boron, Chromium, Copper, Iodine, Iron, Manganese, Molybdenum, Nickel, Silicon, Vanadium, and Zinc*. Washington, DC: National Academy Press.

IOM. 2002/2005. *Dietary Reference Intakes for Energy, Carbohydrate, Fiber, Fat, Fatty Acids, Cholesterol, Protein, and Amino Acids*. Washington, DC: The National Academies Press.

IOM. 2005. *Dietary Reference Intakes for Water, Potassium, Sodium, Chloride, and Sulfate*. Washington, DC: The National Academies Press.

IOM. 2006. *WIC Food Packages: Time for a Change*. Washington, DC: The National Academies Press.

IOM. 2007. *Nutrition Standards for Foods in Schools: Leading the Way Toward Healthier Youth*. Washington, DC: The National Academies Press.

IOM. 2010. *School Meals: Building Blocks for Healthy Children*. Washington, DC: The National Academies Press.

Miech, R. A., S. K. Kumanyika, N. Stettler, B. G. Link, J. C. Phelan, and V. W. Chang. 2006. Trends in the association of poverty with overweight among US adolescents, 1971–2004. *Journal of the American Medical Association* 295(20):2385–2393.

NRC (National Research Council). 1989a. *Diet and Health: Implications for Reducing Chronic Disease Risk*. Washington, DC: National Academy Press.

NRC. 1989b. *Recommended Dietary Allowances*, 10th ed. Washington, DC: National Academy Press.

O'Connor, T. M., S. J. Yang, and T. A. Nicklas. 2006. Beverage intake among preschool children and its effect on weight status. *Pediatrics* 118(4):e1010–e1018.

USDA/FNS (Food and Nutrition Service). 2000. *Building for the Future in the Child and Adult Care Food Program (CACFP)*. http://www.fns.usda.gov/cnd/care/publications/pdf/4Future.pdf (accessed June 29, 2010).

USDA/FNS. 2010. *Program Information Report (Key Data) U.S. Summary, FY 2009–FY 2010*. http://www.fns.usda.gov/fns/key_data/july-2010.pdf (accessed October 19, 2010).

USDA/HHS. 2010. *Report of the Dietary Guidelines Advisory Committee on the Dietary Guidelines for Americans, 2010*. http://www.cnpp.usda.gov/DGAs2010-DGACReport.htm (accessed June 29, 2010).

2

The Child and Adult Care Food Program

The Child and Adult Care Food Program (CACFP) has the broadest scope of any of the U.S. Department of Agriculture (USDA) food programs that specifically target vulnerable populations. In particular, it subsidizes nutritious meals and snacks served to infants and children in participating day care facilities, emergency shelters, and at-risk afterschool programs, and to adults who receive day care in participating facilities. Moreover, a majority of the participants (and many of the providers) are from low-income households. This chapter covers a variety of topics important to the development of revised Meal Requirements. After providing an overview of CACFP, this chapter highlights key elements of the history and growth of the program, describes program settings and clientele, summarizes important aspects of the program's administration and regulations, addresses the program's role in providing a food and nutrition safety net for vulnerable populations, and ends with a brief summary.

PROGRAM OVERVIEW

The goal of CACFP is to serve nutritious meals and snacks to participating children and adults. Ordinarily, the program serves children no older than 12 years of age. However, there are two exceptions: it may serve (1) migrant children ages 15 years and under and (2) youths up to 18 years of age in afterschool programs and in shelters. Adults in participating day care facilities generally are ages 60 years and older. However, individuals from 18 up to 60 years of age may participate if they require daily supervision because of functional limitations.

TABLE 2-1 General Aspects of Current CACFP Meal Requirements

Eating Occasion	Current Requirements
All	Must meet daily pattern, which may differ by age group and setting. The pattern specifies the number of meal components (shown below) and the amount of each.
Breakfast	3 meal components
Lunch or supper	4 meal components
Snacks	Any 2 of 4 components
Meal Component	
Fruit/vegetable	Any fruit and/or vegetable
Grain	Enriched or whole grain
Meat/alternate	None required at breakfast, no restrictions on types
Milk	No restrictions
Food Component	
Energy	No requirement
Micronutrients	No requirement
Fats	No restrictions
Sodium	No restrictions

SOURCE: Adapted from USDA/FNS, 2010a.

To receive reimbursement for the meals and snacks served, participating programs are required to provide meals and snacks according to requirements set by USDA. In this report, the term *meal component* refers to the food groups required in the meals, and the term *food component* refers to nutrients and other substances contained in food. General aspects of the current CACFP Meal Requirements are shown in Table 2-1.

PROGRAM SETTINGS

CACFP is administered in three major types of day care settings, whether for children or adults: family or group homes, centers, and independent centers. The entity responsible for administering the local program depends on the type of setting, as shown in Figure 2-1. Independent centers report directly to the state CACFP agency, whereas other centers and family or group homes must operate under the auspices of a sponsoring organization. A community action agency is a common example of a sponsoring organization. For further information, see the section "Administration and Regulations, Overview."

Sponsoring organizations and independent centers (see Figure 2-1) enter into agreements with their state administering agency to assume administrative and financial responsibility for CACFP operations at the local level, and each state CACFP agency administers the program within the

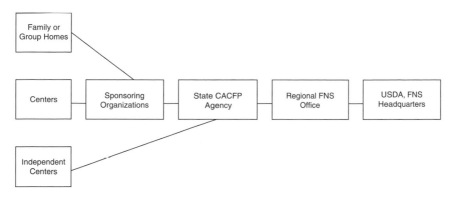

FIGURE 2-1 CACFP settings as administered through USDA FNS.
NOTES: CACFP = Child and Adult Care Food Program; FNS = Food and Nutrition Service; USDA = U.S. Department of Agriculture. All day care homes and
centers must come into the program under a sponsoring organization, which provides training, technical assistance, and monitoring. State CACFP agencies approve
sponsoring organizations and independent centers, monitor the program, provide
guidance, and administer CACFP in most states. USDA FNS administers CACFP at
the federal level through grants to states.
SOURCE: Adapted from USDA/FNS, 2000.

state. Public or private entities that are eligible to participate in CACFP are
described below (USDA/FNS, 2010b).

Day Care Centers for Children and Adults

Child Day Care

Public or private nonprofit child care centers, outside school hours care
centers, Head Start programs, and other institutions that are licensed or
approved to provide day care services are eligible to participate in CACFP,
either independently or as sponsored centers. For-profit centers are eligible
to participate only if, in addition, either (1) they receive title XX funds for
at least 25 percent of enrolled children or licensed capacity (whichever is
less), or (2) at least 25 percent of the children in care are eligible for free
and reduced-price meals. Meals served to children are reimbursed at rates
based upon a child's eligibility for free, reduced-price, or paid meals. In
centers, participants from households with incomes at or below 130 percent
of poverty are eligible for free meals, while those with household incomes
between 130 and 185 percent of poverty are eligible for meals at a reduced
price (USDA/FNS, 2010b).

Adult Day Care

Public or private nonprofit adult day care facilities that provide structured, comprehensive services to nonresident adults who are functionally impaired or ages 60 years and older may participate in CACFP as either independent or sponsored centers. For-profit centers may be eligible for CACFP if at least 25 percent of their participants receive benefits under title XIX or title XX. Meals served to adults receiving care are reimbursed at rates based upon a participant's eligibility for free, reduced-price, or paid meals as defined above (USDA/FNS, 2010b).

Family or Group Day Care Homes for Children

Family or group day care homes (referred to as "homes") are private and must be sponsored by an organization that assumes responsibility for ensuring compliance with federal and state regulations and that acts as a conduit for meal reimbursements to family day care providers. Both family and group day care homes must meet state licensing requirements, where these are imposed, or be approved by a federal, state, or local agency. Group day care homes must be licensed or approved to provide day care services. It is each state's licensing or approval requirements that distinguish a family from a group home.

Homes enroll an average of eight children, including a provider's own children. On average, seven enrolled children are in care in a home on a daily basis. Centers enroll more children than homes. On average, a center that enrolls 60 to 70 children will have 53 to 57 children in attendance daily (USDA/FCS, 1997). Food preparation facilities vary greatly just as kitchens do in homes across the socioeconomic spectrum. Many providers have limited education, but others may have college degrees. In some areas, a substantial number of the providers are not fluent in English. Many providers have incomes at or below the poverty level. The day care home may be a major income source for some providers (USDA/FCS, 1997).

"At-Risk" Afterschool Care Programs

Community-based programs that offer enrichment activities for at-risk children and youth after the regular school day ends may be eligible to provide snacks through CACFP at no cost to the participants. Programs must be offered in areas where at least 50 percent of the children are eligible for free and reduced-price meals based upon school data. Reimbursable suppers are also available to children in eligible afterschool care programs in Connecticut, Delaware, Illinois, Maryland, Michigan, Missouri, Nevada, New York, Oregon, Pennsylvania, Vermont, West Virginia, Wisconsin, and the

District of Columbia (USDA/FNS, 2010b). The effective date of the final rule to add suppers was May 3, 2010 (USDA/FNS, 2010c).

Emergency Shelters

Public or private nonprofit emergency shelters that provide residential and food services to homeless children have been eligible to participate in CACFP since July 1, 1999. Eligible shelters may receive reimbursement for serving up to three meals each day to homeless children, through age 18, who reside there. A shelter does not have to be licensed to provide day care, but it must meet any health and safety codes that are required by state or local law (USDA/FNS, 2010b).

CLIENT CHARACTERISTICS

Age Groups

Section 226.2 of the USDA regulations describes who may receive CACFP meal benefits. Participants must meet the following criteria:

- Children ages 12 years and under, or ages 15 years and under who are children of migrant workers;
- For emergency shelters, persons ages 18 years and under;
- For at-risk afterschool care centers, persons ages 18 years and under at the start of the school year;
- Persons of any age who have one or more disabilities, as determined by the state, and who are enrolled in an institution or child care facility serving a majority of persons who are ages 18 years and under;
- Provider's own children only in a specific low income situation called *tier I* day care homes (see description in the section "Meal Reimbursements") and only when other nonresidential children are enrolled in the day care home and are participating in the meal service; and
- Adult participants who are functionally impaired or 60 years of age or older and who remain in the community (USDA/FNS, 2010b).

HISTORY AND GROWTH OF THE PROGRAM

In 1968, CACFP began as a small 3-year pilot program called the Special Food Service Program for Children. It arose as part of an effort to create an affordable food program for low-income working mothers. Initially, the program provided grants to states to serve meals when schools were not in session. Table 2-2 shows the chronological development and legislative milestones of CACFP. Of special note are (1) the expansion of eligibility, in 1976, to family child care homes that either meet state licensing requirements

TABLE 2-2 Timeline of the Child and Adult Care Food Program

Date	Legislative Action
1968	Public Law (P.L.) 90-302: established the Special Food Service Program for Children (SFSPFC) as a 3-year pilot program
1972	P.L. 92-433: extended the SFSPFC for another 3 years
1975	P.L. 94-105: separated the Child Care Food Program (CCFP) and the Summer Food Service Program
1978	P.L. 95-627: made CCFP permanent
1981	*Omnibus Budget Reconciliation Act of 1981*: amended CCFP reimbursement requirements, reduced reimbursement rates, limited reimbursement, and lowered the maximum age of eligibility through 12 years
1987	*Older Americans Act of 1987*: authorized participation of eligible adult day care centers
1988	*Hunger Prevention Act of 1988*: allowed for a fourth meal for children in care 8 hours or more per day in child care centers and outside school hours centers only
1989	*Child Nutrition and WIC Reauthorization Act of 1989*: changed the name of the program to the Child and Adult Care Food Program (CACFP), funded the expansion of family day care homes into low-income or rural areas, permitted snacks for schools participating in CACFP
1994	*Healthy Meals for Healthy Americans Act of 1994*: extended eligibility for free meals for children participating in Head Start
1996	*Personal Responsibility and Work Opportunity Reconciliation Act of 1996*: replaced the single reimbursement rate with a two-tier structure (two reimbursement rates that consider the provider's economic situation), eliminated reimbursement for a fourth meal, required cost-of-living adjustments for meals served in homes and paid meals served in centers
1998	*Child Nutrition Reauthorization Act of 1998*: authorized CACFP reimbursement for snacks to children through age 18 in afterschool care programs, amended licensing requirements, consolidated benefits for homeless children, reinstated automatic eligibility for free meals for Even Start participants
2000	*Agricultural Risk Protection Act of 2000*: changed eligibility criteria, expanded the at-risk afterschool care component of CACFP
2000	*Consolidated Appropriations Act of 2001*: extended eligibility to for-profit centers and outside of school hours care centers serving low-income children
2001	*Agriculture, Rural Development, FDA, and Related Agencies Appropriations Act of 2002*: authorized supper benefits to some afterschool programs, extended CACFP eligibility to for-profit centers serving low-income children through fiscal year 2002
2004	*Child Nutrition and WIC Reauthorization Act of 2004*: increased the minimum state administrative expense funding; changed the frequency of tiering determination from 3 to 5 years; for military personnel living in privatized housing, excluded counting the household allowance in the determination of eligibility for free and reduced-price meals

NOTE: FDA = Food and Drug Administration; WIC = Special Supplemental Nutrition Program for Women, Infants, and Children.
SOURCE: Adapted from USDA/FNS, 2010d.

or obtain approval from a state or local agency; (2) the provision of financial incentives through P.L. 95-627, in 1978, to expand participation; (3) the change from pilot program status to the permanent Child Care Food Program, also in 1978; and (4) authorization for the adult care component following the enactment of the Older Americans Act of 1987, which resulted in the renaming of the program to the Child and Adult Care Food Program.

CACFP has expanded greatly since its inception as a pilot program (USDA/FNS, 2010d), both in terms of the number of participants served and the types of care programs that are eligible. CACFP currently serves more than 3 million children and adults across the United States and two of its territories: Puerto Rico and Guam. Table 2-3 summarizes key information about program characteristics and program participation and illustrates the diversity of settings and the broad reach of the program.

ADMINISTRATION AND REGULATIONS

Overview

CACFP is authorized by Section 17 of the National School Lunch Act (42 U.S.C. 1766). Regulations for program administration are issued by USDA under 7 C.F.R. Part 226. The CACFP program is administrated by USDA's Food and Nutrition Service through grants to states. At the state level, the state education agency is the usual administrator. In a few states, CACFP is administered by an alternate agency, such as the state health or social services department. The child care component and the adult day care component of CACFP may be administered by different agencies within a state at the discretion of the governor. Independent centers and sponsoring organizations enter into agreements with their administering state agencies to assume administrative and financial responsibility for CACFP operations. Day care homes may participate in the CACFP only under the auspices of a sponsoring organization. Several types of organizations, such as community action agencies and nonprofit organizations, are approved by states to serve as sponsors. Sponsoring organizations provide payment to sponsored day care providers for meals and snacks that meet requirements and are allowed nonfood meal services. The following discussions cover requirements for current meal patterns and key aspects of meal reimbursement.

Current Meal Patterns

CACFP facilities must follow the current meal patterns to receive reimbursement for the meals. The meal patterns for children and adults make use of up to four meal components:

- Fluid milk,
- Fruits/vegetables,

TABLE 2-3 CACFP Program Characteristics and Participation by Provider Type for Fiscal Year 2008, Listed in Descending Order by Average Number of Participants per Month

Provider Type	Participant Characteristics	Licensure	Reimbursement Options	Number of Providers	Number of Participants Served
Child care centers	Children ages 12 years and younger	Licensed or approved	2 meals and 1 snack; or 2 snacks and 1 meal	39,615	1,860,498
Family day care home	Children ages 12 years and younger	Licensed or approved[a]	2 meals and 1 snack; or 2 snacks and 1 meal	141,549	849,568
At-risk afterschool care facility	Children ages 18 years and younger	Approved	1 snack; or 1 snack and 1 meal[b]	6,686	300,008
Outside school hours care facility	Children ages 12 years and younger	Licensed or approved	2 meals and 1 snack	3,131	125,467
Adult care facility	Adults ages 60 years and over and disabled adults	Licensed or approved[c]	2 meals and 1 snack; or 2 snacks and 1 meal	2,568	108,192
Shelters	Children ages 18 years and younger	None	3 meals; or 2 meals and 1 snack	398	7,958

[a]Each state has licensing or approval requirements that distinguish family from group homes and establish maximum participation based on the ratio of infants and children to adults.
[b]At this time, both one snack and one meal are allowed only in 13 states and the District of Columbia.
[c]Dependent on state and local rules for adult day care.
SOURCE: USDA/FNS, 2009.

- Grain/bread, and
- Meat/meat alternates.

As described below, the combination of meal components differs for breakfast, lunch/supper, and snacks; the minimum required amounts of the meal components differ by age group and, for children and adults, by eating occasion.

Meal Pattern Descriptions

Meal patterns for infants differ markedly from those for children and adults, as shown below.

Infants The current infant lunch/supper meal patterns appear in Table 2-4. Ranges are given because of the wide variability in infants' needs based on developmental stage and readiness for foods.

Children and adults For children, a general description of the current minimums required in the meal and snack patterns follows. The general meal pattern description for adults is identical to the list given below except that a serving of milk is not required at supper.

TABLE 2-4 Current Infant Meal Pattern for Lunch or Supper

Food Components	Birth through 3 Months	4–7 Months	8–11 Months
Formula[a] or breast milk[b,c] (fl oz)	4–6	4–8	6–8
Infant cereal[a,d] (T)		0–3[e]	2–4
Fruit or vegetable or both (T)		0–3[e]	1–4
Meat or meat alternate[d]			
Meat, fish, poultry, egg yolk, cooked dry beans or peas (T)			1–4
Cheese (oz)			½–2
Cottage cheese (oz, volume)			1–4
Cheese food or cheese spread (oz, weight)			1–4

NOTE: fl oz = fluid ounce; oz = ounce; T = tablespoon.
[a]Infant formula and dry cereal must be iron-fortified.
[b]Breast milk or formula, or portions of both, may be served; however, breast milk is recommended from birth through 11 months.
[c]For some breastfed infants who regularly consume less than the minimum amount of breast milk per feeding, a serving of less than the minimum amount of breast milk may be offered, with additional breast milk offered if the infant is still hungry.
[d]Menu may include infant cereal, a meat/meat alternate, or both.
[e]A serving of this component is required when the infant is developmentally ready to accept it.
SOURCE: Adapted from USDA/FNS, 2010a.

• Breakfast: one serving each of milk, fruit or vegetable, and grain or bread (three meal components)
• Lunch and Supper: one serving each of milk, grain or bread, meat/meat alternate, and two different servings of fruit or vegetable or a combination of fruit and vegetable (four meal components)
• Snacks: one serving selected from each of two of the four meal components (milk, fruit or vegetable, grain or bread, or meat/meat alternate)—that is, two of the four components.

Serving sizes for children and adults differ by age group, as shown in Table 2-5 for breakfast and in Appendix E for all the other meals and snacks by age group. For children over 12 years of age and adults, the pattern is the same as for children 6–12 years of age with allowance for larger servings. For example, one serving of bread for children ages 1 through 5 years is one-half slice, whereas it is one full slice for children ages 6 through 12 years and may be more for adults. The patterns shown in Table 2-5 and Appendix E include specifications for the types of foods that make up each meal component and the amount of each type of food that represents one serving. Notably, only adult day care centers currently have the option to use the *offer versus serve* form of food service. In this form of service, participants may refuse to take one or more of the meal components offered to them.

By following the breakfast pattern for children 3–5 years of age, a breakfast menu under the current regulations might include one-third cup

TABLE 2-5 Current Child Meal Patterns for Breakfast: Select All Three Meal Components for a Reimbursable Meal

Meal Components	1–2 Years	3–5 Years	6–12 Years[a]
1 Milk (c)	½	¾	1
1 Fruit/vegetable			
Juice,[b] fruit, and/or vegetable (c)	¼	½	½
1 Grain/bread[c]			
Bread (slice)	½	½	1
Cornbread, biscuit, roll, or muffin (svg)	½	½	1
Cold dry cereal (c)	¼	$1/3$	¾
Hot cooked cereal (c)	¼	¼	½
Pasta noodles, or grains (c)	¼	¼	½

NOTE: c = cup; svg = serving.
[a]Children ages 12 years and older may be served larger portions based on their greater needs. They may not be served less than the minimum quantities listed in this column.
[b]Fruit or vegetable juice must be full-strength.
[c]Breads and grains must be made from whole grain or enriched meal or flour. Cereal must be whole grain or enriched or fortified.
SOURCE: Adapted from USDA/FNS, 2010a.

corn flakes with one-half cup sliced banana and three-quarters cup of whole milk (part on the cereal and part in a cup).

The meal components for CACFP were established when the program began in 1968 as the Special Food Service Program for Children. Changes to the regulations for CACFP governing the required meal components in the meal patterns were established by the Personal Responsibility and Work Opportunity Reconciliation Act of 1996 (P.L. 104-193). The mandated changes included a reduction in the number of meals eligible to be claimed for reimbursement to a maximum of two meals and one snack or one meal and two snacks, regardless of the length of time a child was in attendance (see Table 2-3, "Reimbursement Options" column). The CACFP regulations only provide broad nutrient standards for meals or snacks. Useful benchmarks for assessing nutrient standards for CACFP meals and snacks were examined in the Early Childhood and Child Care Study carried out for USDA (USDA/FCS, 1997). These benchmarks came from the school-based programs (7 C.F.R., Parts 210 and 220), which currently call for breakfast to offer at least one-fourth of the Recommended Dietary Allowance (RDA) and for lunch to provide at least one-third of the RDA for these nutrients. Benchmarks for food energy from total fat, saturated fat, and carbohydrate, as well as the total amounts of cholesterol and sodium in the meals and snacks offered, were derived from recommendations in the 1995 *Dietary Guidelines for Americans* (HHS/USDA, 1995) and the *Diet and Health* report (NRC, 1989) (USDA/FCS, 1997).

Meal Reimbursements

Eligible program providers receive reimbursement for meals and snacks served if the meals and foods meet the requirements specified in the regulations (USDA/FNS, 2010a,d,e). The CACFP reimbursement system does not provide partial credit for meals or snacks that meet most of the requirements; they must meet all requirements specified in the meal patterns (see Chapter 7).

Reimbursement Methods

Centers Reimbursement for center-based CACFP facilities is computed by claiming percentages, blended per meal rates, or actual meal count by type (breakfast, lunch, supper, or snack) and considering the eligibility category of participants (free, reduced-price, and paid), which is determined by participant family size and income. As stated above, participants from households with incomes at or below 130 percent of poverty are eligible for free meals. In centers, participants with household incomes between 130 and 185 percent of poverty are eligible for meals at a reduced price (USDA/

FNS, 2010b). The state agency assigns a method of reimbursement for centers, based on meals multiplied by rates, or the lesser of meals multiplied by rates versus actual documented costs. The current reimbursement rates for centers are delineated in Table 2-6; the rates are updated annually.

CACFP centers may operate as pricing or nonpricing programs. Nonpricing programs charge a single fee to cover tuition, meals, and all other day care services; pricing programs charge separate fees for meals. Generally, most CACFP centers, including Head Start programs, operate as nonpricing programs.

TABLE 2-6 Child and Adult Care Food Program (CACFP) Reimbursement Rates per Meal by Meal Type for Adult and Child Day Care Centers, Homes, and Sponsoring Organizations of Day Care Homes, July 1, 2010, through June 30, 2011

		Contiguous States	Alaska	Hawaii
		Whole or Fractions of U.S. Dollars		
Centers				
Breakfast	Paid	0.26	0.39	0.30
	Reduced	1.18	2.06	1.42
	Free	1.48	2.36	1.72
Lunch and supper	Paid	0.26	0.42	0.30
	Reduced	2.32	4.01	2.78
	Free	2.72	4.41	3.18
Snack	Paid	0.06	0.11	0.08
	Reduced	0.37	0.60	0.43
	Free	0.74	1.21	0.87
Day Care Homes				
Breakfast	Tier I[a]	1.19	1.89	1.38
	Tier II[b]	0.44	0.67	0.50
Lunch and supper	Tier I[a]	2.22	3.60	2.60
	Tier II[b]	1.34	2.17	1.57
Snack	Tier I[a]	0.66	1.07	0.77
	Tier II[b]	0.18	0.29	0.21

NOTE: These rates do not include the value of commodities (or cash in lieu of commodities) that some facilities receive as additional assistance for each lunch or supper served to participants under CACFP. The national average minimum value of donated food, or cash in lieu thereof, per lunch and supper under CACFP (7 C.F.R. Part 226) will be 20.25 cents for the period July 1, 2010, through June 30, 2011 (USDA/FNS, 2010f).

[a]Tier I homes are those located in low-income areas or run by providers with family incomes at or below 185 percent of the federal poverty guideline (USDA/FNS, 1997).

[b]Tier II homes are those that do not meet either the location- or provider-income criterion for a tier I home (USDA/FNS, 1997).

SOURCE: Adapted from USDA/FNS, 2010e.

Day care homes The Personal Responsibility and Work Opportunity Reconciliation Act of 1996 (P.L. 104-193) refocused the family child care component of CACFP on low-income children by establishing a two-tier system of reimbursement rates for family child care homes. Tier I day care homes are those that are located in low-income areas, or those in which the provider's household income is at or below 185 percent of the federal income poverty guidelines. Tier II homes are those family day care homes that do not meet either the location- or provider-income criterion for a tier I home.

Sponsoring organizations may use elementary school free and reduced-price enrollment data or census block group data to determine which areas are low income. However, the provider in a tier II home may elect to have the sponsoring organization identify income-eligible children. When this is done, the meals served to children who qualify for free and reduced-price meals are reimbursed at the higher tier I rates. Program payments for day care homes are based on the number of approved meals served to enrolled children multiplied by the appropriate reimbursement rate (tier I or tier II; see above) for each breakfast, lunch, supper, or snack.

MONITORING THE QUALITY OF CACFP MEALS

Current federal regulations require that state agencies annually conduct monitoring reviews of at least one-third of all CACFP institutions[1] and must follow a specific review cycle for sponsors and their sponsored centers and day care homes, with the number of homes monitored based on the home sponsor. The state may conduct additional reviews and/or provide technical assistance for those institutions that need close observation. The purpose of the monitoring is to examine the extent to which the institutions are complying with the CACFP requirements. States monitor the entire CACFP operation, including the ability of child care providers to adequately plan, prepare, and serve a reimbursable meal and to provide nutrition education to its participants. To ensure that the institution meets the CACFP requirements, state monitors also review the institution's financial viability and financial management systems, internal controls, and other management practices and systems.

Indicators of compliance include record keeping; meal counts; menus; licensing and approval; production records, where applicable; meal observation; administrative costs; and, for sponsor organizations, training and monitoring of their sponsored facilities. States provide technical assistance

---

[1]As defined in federal CACFP regulations at 7 C.F.R. 226.2, "institution means a sponsoring organization, child care center, at-risk afterschool care center, outside-school-hours care center, emergency shelter or adult day care center which enters into an agreement with the State agency to assume final administrative and financial responsibility for Program operations."

as needed, and many combine the monitoring and technical assistance visits. Generally the review covers a specific test month. If further evaluation is warranted, other months may be combined in the review. The state may require the CACFP institutions to develop and submit written corrective action plans to improve and permanently correct any program violations noted during the visit in order to achieve compliance with requirements. If meal deficiencies are observed during the evaluation of the menus (and production records where applicable) and the meal observation, the state may disallow (not reimburse) meals. Because many CACFP institutions have had difficulty completing and maintaining production records that provide enough data to substantiate the validity of the meals produced, several states have eliminated the production record-keeping requirement. In its place, they use receipts and invoices to support the meal reimbursement claims.

CACFP AS PART OF THE FOOD AND NUTRITION SAFETY NET

CACFP is one of 15 nutrition assistance programs administered by the FNS of USDA. These programs provide a safety net for low-income individuals and specific groups that may be vulnerable to social and environmental factors that place them at increased nutritional risk. Of special note, children who consume meals offered through CACFP may also consume food provided through other established nutrition programs such as the Supplemental Nutrition Program for Women, Infants, and Children or through the School Breakfast Program (SBP) and the National School Lunch Program (NSLP). Because these are very large programs that serve millions of the nation's children, it will be especially useful for the CACFP Meal Requirements to align well with the foods and nutrition education provided by these programs.

A new and much smaller program recently introduced by the FNS is the Fresh Fruit and Vegetable Program, which began as a pilot program in 4 states and is now a nation-wide program in selected schools in all 50 states, the District of Columbia, Guam, Puerto Rico, and the Virgin Islands. This program provides fresh fruits and vegetables to low-income children, who may also receive meals through CACFP (USDA/FNS, 2010g). Appendix F contains brief descriptions of most of these programs and identifies websites that provide more detailed information.

CACFP serves a key role in the U.S. food and nutrition safety net. As such, CACFP is expected to meet a portion of participants' nutritional needs and to be in alignment with current nutrition policy and guidance, including the current *Dietary Guidelines for Americans* (HHS/USDA, 2005) and Dietary Reference Intakes. The following briefly addresses concerns about food insecurity in today's environment and summarizes CACFP's potential contribution to the nutrition of individuals in day care.

Concerns About Food Insecurity

Food insecurity, the uncertainty of having enough food to meet the basic needs of household members, places children at risk for inadequate food and nutrient intake and for impaired or diminished growth. Among both children and adults, food insecurity increases the risk for behavioral and psychosocial dysfunction (Miller et al., 2008) and poor health outcomes, including infant and toddler development (Biros et al., 2005; Kirkpatrick et al., 2010; Rose-Jacobs et al., 2008; Stuff et al., 2004). The monitoring of food insecurity across the nation by USDA indicates that, as of 2007, the prevalence of food insecurity among children was 8.3 percent and was 11.1 percent for households (USDA/ERS, 2009a). By the end of 2008, the prevalence of household food insecurity had increased to 14.6 percent, the highest prevalence since data collection began in 1995 (USDA/ERS, 2009b).

A high proportion of children served by CACFP can be considered vulnerable to food insecurity because they are from low-income households. However, economic status alone does not predict "hunger" or food insecurity. Adult participants may be vulnerable to food insecurity for another reason: functional impairments may limit their ability to obtain, store, and prepare enough food to meet their needs. Taken together, the population served by CACFP may be considered at higher risk for food insecurity and its associated outcomes than the general population.

Potential Impact of CACFP on Client's Food and Nutrient Intake

Considering the U.S. population as a whole, CACFP makes a much greater contribution to the food and nutrient intakes of the nation's children, especially its young children, than it does to its adults. The potential impact of CACFP on individuals in day care settings that participate in the program, whether children or adults, depends on the number of hours spent in day care and thus the amount of food they are served. The discussion below covers participation in day care and the potential contribution of calories from meals served during day care.

Child Care Participation

Overview The document *America's Children: Key National Indicators of Well-Being* estimates that 36 percent of the U.S. child population ages 0–6 years are cared for in center-based programs that include child care centers,

Head Start programs, publicly funded pre-kindergarten, and private child care (Federal Interagency Forum on Child and Family Statistics, 2009).

As discussed in Chapter 1, family day care homes and traditional child care centers comprise the majority of CACFP providers (more than 93 percent). Preschool children, the largest age group in full-day care, were reported by the U.S. Census Bureau to spend about 32 hours per week in care of any type. According to the 2006 *Survey of Income and Program Participation*, the number of children younger than 5 years of age reported in all child care arrangements in the United States was about 12.7 million (U.S. Census Bureau, 2006).

Ethnic and socioeconomic considerations   Data from the U.S. Census Bureau indicate there are substantial ethnic and socioeconomic differences among children enrolled in different types of day care programs. Enrollment data from 2004 by racial and ethnic group showed that about 25 percent of black, Asian, and non-Hispanic white children of working mothers were enrolled in day care. By comparison, only 5 percent of children of Hispanic working mothers were enrolled in day care. Hispanic mothers were twice as likely as non-Hispanic white mothers to rely on relatives, including siblings, for care of their preschool children (19 vs. 7 percent, respectively; U.S. Census Bureau, 2006). Enrollment in day care programs is 10 percent greater for children from families with incomes above the federal poverty level than for children from families in poverty, whose children are more likely to be cared for by a sibling (U.S. Census Bureau, 2006).

Meals in day care   Child day care homes provided 497.5 million meals in fiscal year (FY) 2010 and child day care centers provided 1.1 billion meals during that same period (USDA/FNS, 2010h, Table 13a). The committee was unable to locate current program-wide data on average meals served to participants per unit of time by age group. To try to provide some perspective, the very limited available information on CACFP's contribution to children's nutrition is summarized below.

Analysis of survey data gathered in 1999 from parents or guardians of children served by CACFP family day care homes found that children in tier II homes would likely consume 50 percent of their daily energy requirements from the breakfast-lunch-one-snack-meal combination and two-thirds from the breakfast-lunch-two-snack-combination (USDA/ERS, 2002).

Children in afterschool programs, who are typically in care for a minimum of 2 hours a day, generally receive only one snack—a small fraction of their daily food needs. These participants, however, may have been provided slightly more than half of their daily food needs through the SBP and the NSLP combined. Those children in the afterschool programs that are allowed to receive supper in addition to a snack would be expected to receive roughly one-third of their daily calorie requirements from CACFP.

Adult Day Care Participation

According to the National Adult Day Services Association, 3,500 adult day care facilities across the United States are caring for approximately 150,000 adults daily (Robert Wood Johnson Foundation, 2007). USDA surveys indicate that adult day care centers provided 56 million meals to participants in FY 2010 (USDA/FNS, 2010h, Table 15b). Based on the current CACFP meal pattern, adults in day care have the opportunity to meet approximately two-thirds of their calorie needs while attending adult day care centers that provide CACFP services.

SUMMARY

To contribute to the health of persons in day care, the Child and Adult Care Food Program subsidizes the cost of nutritious meals and snacks to participating independent day care centers and, through sponsoring organizations, to other centers and day care homes. More than 3 million children and adults are served through CACFP yearly. To receive reimbursement for the foods served, participating sites are required to provide meals and snacks that meet minimum requirements. The current requirements specify which meal components (fruit/vegetables, grains, meat/meat alternates, milk) must be included in the meals and snacks and the minimum amounts of each. Especially for the infants, children, and adults that are in day care for much of the day, CACFP provides a large majority of their daily food and nutrient intake and makes a major contribution to the food and nutrition safety net.

REFERENCES

Biros, M. H., P. L. Hoffman, and K. Resch. 2005. The prevalence and perceived health consequences of hunger in emergency department patient populations. *Academic Emergency Medicine* 12(4):310–317.

Federal Interagency Forum on Child and Family Statistics. 2009. *America's Children: Key National Indicators of Well-Being, 2009*. Washington, DC: U.S. Government Printing Office. http://www.childstats.gov/pdf/ac2009/ac_09.pdf (accessed September 28, 2010).

HHS/USDA. 1995. *Nutrition and Your Health: Dietary Guidelines for Americans*. Washington, DC: U.S. Government Printing Office. http://www.health.gov/DIETARYGUIDELINES/dga95/default.htm (accessed December 16, 2010).

HHS/USDA (U.S. Department of Health and Human Services/U.S. Department of Agriculture). 2005. *Dietary Guidelines for Americans*, 6th ed. Washington, DC: U.S. Government Printing Office. http://www.health.gov/DietaryGuidelines/dga2005/document/ (accessed July 23, 2008).

Kirkpatrick, S. I., L. McIntyre, and M. L. Potestio. 2010. Child hunger and long-term adverse consequences for health. *Archives of Pediatrics and Adolescent Medicine* 164(8):754–762.

Miller, E., K. M. Wieneke, J. M. Murphy, S. Desmond, A. Schiff, K. M. Canenguez, and R. E. Kleinman. 2008. Child and parental poor health among families at risk for hunger attending a community health center. *Journal of Health Care for the Poor and Underserved* 19(2):550–561.

NRC (National Research Council). 1989. *Diet and Health: Implications for Reducing Chronic Disease Risk.* Washington, DC: National Academy Press.

Robert Wood Johnson Foundation. 2007. *National Adult Day Services Association Becomes Independent Organization, Expands Outreach through New Materials, Conferences and Member Hotline.* http://www.rwjf.org/reports/grr/040623.htm (accessed August 11, 2010).

Rose-Jacobs, R., M. M. Black, P. H. Casey, J. T. Cook, D. B. Cutts, M. Chilton, T. Heeren, S. M. Levenson, A. F. Meyers, and D. A. Frank. 2008. Household food insecurity: Associations with at-risk infant and toddler development. *Pediatrics* 121(1):65–72.

Stuff, J. E., P. H. Casey, K. L. Szeto, J. M. Gossett, J. M. Robbins, P. M. Simpson, C. Connell, and M. L. Boglet. 2004. Household food insecurity is associated with adult health status. *Journal of Nutrition* 134(9):2330–2335.

U.S. Census Bureau. 2006. *Survey of Income and Program Participation.* http://www.census.gov/sipp/index.html (accessed July 11, 2010).

USDA/ERS (Economic Research Service). 2002. *Households with Children in CACFP Child Care Homes—Effects of Meal Reimbursement Tiering: A Report to Congress on the Family Child Care Homes Legislative Changes Study.* Washington, DC: USDA/ERS. http://www.ers.usda.gov/publications/efan02002/efan02002.pdf (accessed October 11, 2010).

USDA/ERS. 2009a. *Food Insecurity in Households with Children: Prevalence, Severity, and Household Characteristics.* Washington, DC: USDA/ERS. http://www.ers.usda.gov/publications/eib56/eib56.pdf (accessed March 25, 2010).

USDA/ERS. 2009b. *Household Food Security in the United States, 2008.* Washington, DC: USDA/ERS. http://www.ers.usda.gov/publications/err83/err83.pdf (accessed September 27, 2010).

USDA/FCS (Food and Consumer Service). 1997. *Early Childhood and Child Care Study: Nutritional Assessment of the CACFP: Final Report, Volume 2.* Alexandria, VA: USDA/FCS. http://www.fns.usda.gov/ora/menu/Published/CNP/cnp-archive.htm (accessed July 9, 2010).

USDA/FNS (Food and Nutrition Service). 1997. Child and Adult Care Food Program; Improved Targeting of Day Care Home Reimbursements. *Federal Register* 62(4):889–915.

USDA/FNS. 2000. *Building for the Future in the Child and Adult Care Food Program (CACFP).* http://www.fns.usda.gov/cnd/care/publications/pdf/4Future.pdf (accessed June 29, 2010).

USDA/FNS. 2009. *Child and Adult Care Food Program: Building for the Future.* PowerPoint presentation at the open session of the IOM committee on December 8, Washington, DC.

USDA/FNS. 2010a. *Child and Adult Care Food Program Meal Patterns.* http://www.fns.usda.gov/cnd/care/Program Basics/Meals/Meal_Patterns.htm (accessed March 24, 2010).

USDA/FNS. 2010b. *Child and Adult Care Food Program.* http://www.fns.usda.gov/cnd/care/cacfp/aboutcacfp.htm (accessed July 9, 2010).

USDA/FNS. 2010c. Child and Adult Care Food Program: At-Risk Afterschool Meals in Eligible State. *Federal Register* 75(62):16325–16325.

USDA/FNS. 2010d. *Child and Adult Care Food Program Legislative History.* http://www.fns.usda.gov/cnd/Care/Regs-Policy/Legislation/history.htm (accessed March 24, 2010).

USDA/FNS. 2010e. Child and Adult Care Food Program: National Average Payment Rates, Day Care Home Food Service Payment Rates, and Administrative Reimbursement Rates for Sponsoring Organizations of Day Care Homes for the Period July 1, 2010 Through June 30, 2011. *Federal Register* 75(137):41793–41795.

USDA/FNS. 2010f. Food Distribution Program: Value of Donated Foods From July 1, 2010 Through June 30, 2011. *Federal Register* 75(137):41795.

USDA/FNS. 2010g. *Fresh Fruit and Vegetable Program.* http://www.fns.usda.gov/cnd/FFVP/FFVPdefault.htm (accessed March 24, 2010).

USDA/FNS. 2010h. *Program Information Report (Key Data) U.S. Summary, FY 2009–FY 2010.* http://www.fns.usda.gov/fns/key_data/july-2010.pdf (accessed October 19, 2010).

3

Methods for Examining Food and Nutrient Intakes

The committee examined the dietary intakes of food groups, food subgroups, and nutrients by infants, children, and adults to identify food and nutrient intakes needing improvement for each of the identified age groups of Child and Adult Care Food Program (CACFP) participants. This chapter briefly covers the data sources used along with their strengths and limitations, the standards against which intakes were measured, and the methods used to examine food and nutrient intakes.

FOOD AND NUTRIENT DATA SOURCES

Brief Description

The primary source of data on food and nutrient intake was the *What We Eat in America* component of the National Health and Nutrition Examination Survey (NHANES) 2003–2004. These specific survey years were selected as the most complete source of data on the nutrients and food groups of interest. NHANES is conducted by the National Center for Health Statistics and is designed to provide national estimates of the health and nutrition status of the civilian, noninstitutionalized population in the 50 states. The data used included dietary intake data on individuals of all ages; demographic information including age, gender, and physiological status (e.g., whether a woman was pregnant or lactating); and measures of stature and weight by age. Data on supplement use were not included in the analyses. All analyses used the appropriate statistical weights to adjust for the NHANES sample design. For the estimation of variances of quantities of interest, the committee used the method of balanced repeated replication and constructed the replicated weight sets as described by Fuller (2009).The main data source for food group intake was the MyPyramid Equivalents Database, 2.0 (MPED 2.0), for U.S. Department of Agriculture (USDA) Survey Foods, 2003–2004. This database translates the amounts of foods reported in the dietary recalls from the *What We Eat in America* survey (USDA/ARS, 2004) into the number of equivalents for each of the 32 major food groups and subgroups in MyPyramid. The MPED 2.0 includes variables for discretionary solid fat (including some oils), added sugars, and alcoholic beverages.

Data on vitamin D were obtained from *What We Eat in America*, NHANES 2007–2008 (USDA/ARS, 2010a, Table 1). Limited food intake data were also available from the first Feeding Infants and Toddlers Study (FITS) (Ziegler et al., 2006). The FITS survey population included a large, representative, cross-sectional sample of parents or caregivers that provided information on the diet and eating habits of infants, toddlers, and preschoolers living in the United States. Its primary objective was to obtain information on nutrient intakes and gaps, and consumption patterns within this population. The first FITS was conducted in 2002, and the second FITS was initiated in 2008 and completed in 2009. The second survey included an expanded sample size and age range of 0 to 48 months (Nestlé Nutrition Institute, 2009), but data from the second survey were not available to the committee.

Strengths and Limitations

Strengths of the NHANES 2003–2004 data sets relate to the survey design, quality control, large sample size, and availability of data on nutrients of interest to the committee. Limitations relate to the lack of reliable data on supplement intake (mentioned above); the accuracy of the self-reported dietary intakes (diet recalls); and, for the purposes of this report, the relatively small number of low-income infants, children, and adults.

Self-Reported Dietary Data

The under-reporting of food intakes appears to be more common than over-reporting at all age levels including children and adolescents, and especially among persons who are overweight or obese (Braam et al., 1998; Bratteby et al., 1998; Fisher et al., 2000; Little et al., 1999). There is further evidence that psychological factors contribute to under-reporting, and these may be more prevalent among obese women (Kretsch et al., 1999; Scagliusi et al., 2003). The accuracy of dietary reporting, particularly that related to children, however, is highly dependent on the survey instrument (Livingstone and Robson, 2000).

The NHANES dietary data used by the committee were obtained using the Automated Multiple-Pass Method, which limits the under-reporting of food intakes (Johnson et al., 2008) and improves the accuracy of estimated energy intakes in normal-weight adults (Moshfegh et al., 2008). Even using this method, however, Moshfegh and colleagues (2008) found that individuals who were overweight or obese under-reported their intakes. Although the under-reporting of energy is reasonably well documented, the extent to which nutrients are underestimated is unclear. Results obtained in the Observing Protein and Energy Nutrition study conducted by the National Cancer Institute (Subar et al., 2003) suggest that individuals who under-report do so for all food groups, but the degree of under-reporting can vary between foods. The implication of the under-reporting of food intakes is an overestimation of the prevalence of inadequacy; that is, more of the individuals may have adequate intakes than the analysis indicates. The over-reporting of food intake may be most likely for young children (up to about age 8 years) (Basch et al., 1990; Lytle et al., 1993). The major implication of the over-reporting of food intake is that the prevalence of nutrient inadequacy may be underestimated.

Number of Low-Income Subjects

Because the sample sizes for low-income individuals were small and would not provide reliable data about intakes at the tails of the intake distribution, the committee considered the extent of the difference by income. Using weighted 1-day dietary intake data from *What We Eat in America*, NHANES 2003–2004, for individuals ages 2 years and over (USDA/ARS, 2010b, Table 7), the committee compared mean intakes of calories and selected nutrients for those with incomes below 185 percent of the federal poverty level and those with higher incomes. Calorie intakes were similar (2,183 vs. 2,204 kcal/d for those with lower vs. higher incomes). Looking specifically at children ages 2 through 5 years, nutrient intakes tended to be somewhat higher for the lower-income children (for example, iron intakes were 13.9 mg/d vs. 11.3 mg/d for the higher-income children). Thus, nutrients of concern for the full sample would encompass those of concern for the low-income sample. Based on these findings, the committee considered it appropriate to use the data spanning the entire income range in order to increase the reliability of the intake estimates.

Despite the limitations addressed above, the dietary intake data were an important source of information for examining food and nutrient intakes. These data enabled the committee to identify nutrients likely to be either under- or overconsumed by the age groups examined.

STANDARDS USED TO REVIEW FOOD INTAKES

Infants and Children Younger Than 2 Years of Age

Because the *Dietary Guidelines for Americans* (HHS/USDA, 2005) excludes children under the age of 2 years, published statements of the American Academy of Pediatrics (AAP) were used as the source of dietary guidance for this age group (see Table 3-1). Nutrient intakes were examined using Dietary Reference Intakes (see later section "Nutrient Intake Evaluation").

The AAP acknowledges that there is little evidence for order of first foods and states that its preferred first foods are iron-fortified cereal and pureed meat (AAP, 2009). However because iron and zinc are better absorbed from meat than grains, they may be a preferred first food, particularly for breastfed infants (Krebs et al., 2006).

Children Over 2 Years of Age and Adults

The standard used to review food intakes of persons over 2 years of age was the MyPyramid food guidance system.[1] MyPyramid provides specific food-based dietary guidance that are consistent with the recommendations in the 2005 *Dietary Guidelines for Americans* (HHS/USDA, 2005) for all individuals over the age of 2 years. That is, MyPyramid uses food patterns to translate the 2005 *Dietary Guidelines* into recommendations about the types and amounts of food that will promote health and healthy weight (Marcoe et al., 2006). Extensive information about MyPyramid is available online at www.mypyramid.gov. A key aspect of MyPyramid concerns the forms of foods used to develop the food patterns. In particular, the foods included in each of the MyPyramid food groups are the lowest in fat (e.g., lean meat and fat-free milk), and they are free of added sugars (e.g., water-packed canned fruit).

THE DETERMINATION OF AGE GROUPS, BODY WEIGHTS AND HEIGHTS, AND ESTIMATED CALORIE REQUIREMENTS

Before dietary intakes could be assessed, it was necessary to establish appropriate age groups for CACFP, determine body weights and heights by

---

[1]The DASH diet eating plan (NHLBI, 2010; http://www.nhlbi.nih.gov/hbp/prevent/h_eating/h_eating.htm), which is very similar to the MyPyramid food guide, has been documented to lower blood pressure among adults (Appel et al., 2006; Ard et al., 2004; Sacks et al., 2001); however the committee found that its use for review of food intakes and planning meals for CACFP would present logistical problems. For example, it would not match satisfactorily with the MyPyramid Equivalents Database, 2.0, for USDA Survey Foods, 2003–2004 (MPED 2.0).

TABLE 3-1 Dietary Guidance for Infants and Children Under the Age of 2 Years

Dietary Guidance	Source
Breastfeeding	
Breastfeeding is the preferred method of infant feeding because of the nutritional value and health benefits of human milk.	AAP, 2005, 2009
Encourage breastfeeding with exclusion of other foods until infants are around 6 months of age.	AAP, 2005, 2009; WHO, 2002, 2003
Continue breastfeeding for first year after birth.	AAP, 2005, 2009
Continue breastfeeding into second year after birth if mutually desired by the mother and child.	AAP, 2001a, 2005, 2009; Kleinman, 2000
Formula Feeding	
For infants who are not currently breastfeeding, use infant formula throughout the first year after birth.	AAP, 2001a, 2005, 2009; Kleinman, 2000
Infant formula used during the first year after birth should be iron-fortified.	AAP, 1999, 2001a, 2005, 2009
Feeding Other Foods to Infants and Young Children	
Introduce semisolid complementary foods gradually beginning around 6 months of age.	AAP, 2005, 2009; Kleinman, 2000; WHO, 2002, 2003
Introduce single-ingredient complementary foods, one at a time for a several-day trial.	AAP, 2009
Introduce a variety of semisolid complementary foods throughout ages 6–12 months.	AAP, 2009; WHO, 2003
Encourage consumption of iron-rich complementary foods during ages 6–12 months.	AAP, 2001b, 2005, 2009
Avoid introducing fruit juice before 6 months of age.	AAP, 2001b, 2009; Kleinman, 2000
Limit intake of fruit juice to 4–6 fluid ounces/day for children ages 1–6 years.	AAP, 2001b, 2009
Encourage children to eat whole fruits to meet their recommended daily fruit intake.	AAP, 2001b, 2009
Delay the introduction of cow's milk until the second year after birth.	AAP, 2005, 2009
Cow's milk fed during the second year after birth (age 1 year) should be whole milk.	AAP, 2009
Developing Healthy Eating Patterns	
Provide children with repeated exposure to new foods to optimize acceptance and encourage development of eating habits that promote selection of a varied diet.	AAP, 2009; ADA, 2004
Prepare complementary foods without added sugars or salt (i.e., sodium).	AAP, 2009
Promote healthy eating early in life.	ADA, 2004
Promoting Food Safety	
Avoid feeding hard, small, particulate foods up to age 4 years to reduce risk of choking.	AAP, 2009

age group, and estimate calorie requirements by age group. These topics are addressed below.

Establishing Age Groups

Throughout the report, the committee uses the notation X–Y to mean X *through* Y months or years (e.g., 2–4 years means ages 2 through 4 years and 11 months). One of the first steps in the committee's approach was to establish age groups to use to examine food and nutrient intakes. Current CACFP regulations specify requirements for infants, three groups of children (1–2, 3–5, and 6–12 years), and adults. However, the committee selected different age ranges to evaluate children's and adults' intakes relative to current dietary guidance. Descriptive data on food group and nutrient intakes were *initially* calculated for the following age groups:

- Infants ages 6–11 months;
- Preschool children age 1 year;
- Preschool children ages 2–4 years;
- Schoolchildren ages 5–10 years;
- Schoolchildren ages 11–13 years;
- Youth ages 14–18 years;
- Adults ages 19–59 years;
- Older adults ages 60 years and older; and
- Older adults ages 70 years and older.

The age groups for children were chosen to conform with (1) the ages used by the Committee to Review the WIC Food Packages (IOM, 2006a) for preschool children and (2) those used by the Committee on Nutrition Standards for the National School Lunch and Breakfast Program (IOM, 2010) for schoolchildren and adolescents.

For infants, analyses were not performed for those under 6 months of age because intakes from breast milk could not be quantified. However, because breast milk is a poor source of iron and zinc after 6 months of age, intakes of these two nutrients were examined by breastfeeding status for infants 6–11 months of age.

Separate analyses were performed for younger adults (ages 19–59 years) and adults 60 years of age and older because of differences in their calorie requirements. Initial analyses compared the intakes of adults ages 60 years and older with those of adults ages 70 years and older. The differences were not large, however, and only the broader age group (60 years and older) was used for further analyses.

The relatively few pregnant and lactating women were not excluded from the analyses, nor were their intakes examined separately. Because very few pregnant and lactating women are likely to participate in the adult care portion of CACFP, their requirements were not considered separately. Their nutrient needs would be somewhat higher than those for most women.

Determination of Body Weights and Heights

Body weight is used to estimate both calorie requirements and protein requirements, and height (length for infants and young children) is also needed to estimate calorie requirements. Therefore, the mean and median body weights and heights were calculated for each age group using anthropometric measures from NHANES 2003–2004. Table 3-2 shows the results by gender and age group.

Estimation of Calorie Requirements

To compare food group intakes with those recommended by MyPyramid, it was necessary to select an appropriate MyPyramid pattern for each age group. Because the patterns are determined by calorie requirements, an estimation of calorie needs was made for each CACFP age group, based on

TABLE 3-2 Calculated Mean and Median Body Weights and Heights by Age Group Based on NHANES 2003–2004

Age and Gender Group	Mean Body Weight (kg)	Median Body Weight (kg)	Mean Height (cm)	Median Height (cm)
1 year	11.6	11.5	82.2[a]	81.8[a]
2–4 years	16.1	15.9	99.2	99.1
5–10 years				
Males	30.6	28.5	129.1	129.1
Females	31.2	27.9	129.5	128.9
11–13 years				
Males	54.3	51.8	157.5	156.7
Females	53.6	51.4	155.7	155.6
14–18 years				
Males	73.0	69.7	174.7	175.2
Females	63.2	59.5	161.9	161.9
19–59 years				
Males	88.0	85.7	177.0	177.3
Females	75.3	70.7	163.1	163.1
≥ 60 years				
Males	87.3	85.5	174.7	174.8
Females	73.0	70.3	160.4	160.1

NOTE: kg = kilogram; NA = not applicable; NHANES = National Health and Nutrition Examination Survey.
[a]Recumbent lengths are given for children 1 year old.
SOURCE: NHANES 2003–2004.

the age- and gender-specific Estimated Energy Requirement (EER) equations in *Dietary Reference Intakes: Energy, Carbohydrate, Fiber, Fat, Fatty Acids, Cholesterol, Protein, and Amino Acids* (IOM, 2002/2005). In addition, for children 2 years and older and adults, the committee specified a physical activity level (PAL). The values selected are either low-active or active for the children and sedentary for the adults, as summarized below:

- For children ages 1 year and 2–4 years, the committee adopted the approach used by the Committee to Review the WIC Food Packages (IOM, 2006a). This included the use of median heights and weights described in the Dietary Reference Intakes report that includes the EER equations (IOM, 2002/2005) and, for children 2–4 years, a low-active PAL.
- For children ages 5–10, 11–13, and 14–18 years, the committee adopted the approach used by the Committee on Nutrition Standards for the National School Lunch and Breakfast Program (IOM, 2010). This included the use of median heights and weights from the Centers for Disease Control and Prevention (CDC) growth charts (Kuczmarski et al., 2000), an active PAL for children 5–10 years, and a low-active PAL for children and adolescents 11–18 years.
- For adults 19 years and older, the committee used heights and selected weights from NHANES 2003–2004 and a sedentary PAL. Because a large portion of the adult NHANES population is overweight, actual weights were not used. Instead, for adults ages 19–59 years, actual weights were replaced with weights that would be consistent with a body mass index (BMI) of 22 (as a midpoint within the range of recommended BMI) for actual heights. For adults ages 60 years and older, the weights used were consistent with a BMI of 25 for actual heights. The use of the higher BMI for this age group was based on evidence that a proportion of the disabled population requiring day care may be at greater risk of low energy intake (Bartali et al., 2003; Sharkey, 2008).

Estimated EERs are shown in Table 3-3 by age group and gender and by age group for males and females combined.

FOOD INTAKE EVALUATION

The evaluation of food intake tends to be complex because many foods are consumed episodically rather than regularly. As described in Appendix G, only one of two possible approaches to use was considered feasible. The Iowa State University Foods method (Nusser et al., 1996) was tested

TABLE 3-3 Median and Mean Estimated Energy Requirements (EERs) and Rounded Calorie Levels by Age Group

Age Group (years)	Median or Mean[a] Calorie Level			Rounded Calorie Levels for Males and Females
	Males	Females	Average of Males and Females	
1	NA	NA	935	950
2–4	NA	NA	1,285	1,300
5–10	1,894	1,765	1,830	1,800
11–13	2,125	1,905	2,015	2,000
14–18	2,686	2,044	2,365	2,400
19–29[a]	2,725	2,078	2,401	2,400
30–39[a]	2,636	2,046	2,341	2,300
40–49[a]	2,567	1,997	2,282	2,300
50–59[a]	2,489	1,920	2,204	2,200
≥ 60[a]	2,209	1,687	1,948	1,900

NOTE: NA = not applicable.

[a]Calorie levels for adults ≥ 19 years are mean EERs.

SOURCES: EERs for 1 and 2–4 years were calculated based on data from the Continuing Survey of Food Intakes by Individuals (USDA/ARS, 2000) using the median heights method described in the Dietary Reference Intake report (IOM, 2002/2005), as shown in IOM (2006a, p. 51). EERs for 5–10, 11–13, and 14–18 years were calculated using median height and weight from CDC growth charts (Kuczmarski et al., 2000), as shown in IOM (2010, p. 70). EERs for adults over age 19 were calculated using data from NHANES 2003–2004.

and found appropriate to use to estimate usual food intakes. Mean calorie intakes from discretionary solid fat and added sugars were estimated using the values 9 calories per gram of fat and 4 calories per gram of sugar. To evaluate how well children's and adult's usual food group intakes aligned with *Dietary Guidelines for Americans*, the committee compared the mean food group intakes for one day with the MyPyramid food patterns (USDA, 2009) for the selected age groups and calorie levels. Calories from solid fat and added sugars were compared with MyPyramid's allowance for calories from these sources. Tables of the comparisons appear in Chapter 4 (Table 4-1) and Chapter 5 (Table 5-1).

NUTRIENT INTAKE EVALUATION

A primary focus of the committee's assessment of nutrients was to examine the apparent prevalence of inadequate or excessive intakes of nutrients. To carry out the intake assessments, the committee estimated usual nutrient intakes and used methods recommended and described by the Institute of Medicine (IOM) for the assessment of energy and nutrient intakes (IOM, 2000). These methods make use of the Estimated Average

Requirement (EAR), Adequate Intake (AI), and Tolerable Upper Intake Level (UL), but not the Recommended Dietary Allowance (RDA). The methods used in estimating usual intakes and applying the different types of reference values are described below and in Appendix G.

Estimating Usual Nutrient Intakes

The usual intake of a nutrient is an individual's long-term average intake of that nutrient (NRC, 1986). Usual intake must be estimated; it cannot be observed, because day-to-day intakes vary considerably. The Iowa State University method (Nusser et al., 1996) is the commonly used and accepted approach for estimating the usual intakes by population groups. This method estimates the distribution of usual intakes by using a single 24-hour recall for all members of the group and a second 24-hour recall for some proportion of the group. For NHANES 2003–2004, a second 24-hour recall was collected for all persons in the sample. The personal computer version of the Software for Intake Distribution Estimation (PC-SIDE; ISU, 1997) was used to estimate (1) usual nutrient intake distributions and (2) the proportion of children and adults with usual intakes above or below the defined cutoff values.

Applying the Dietary Reference Intakes:
Institute of Medicine Methodology

The Dietary Reference Intakes (DRIs) released by the IOM replaced the previously used RDAs (NRC, 1989) as authoritative reference values. The DRIs provide several types of reference values for use in the assessment and planning of diets of groups, including the EAR, the AI for nutrients without an EAR, the UL, and the Acceptable Macronutrient Distribution Range (AMDR). Definitions of these DRIs are given in Box 3-1.

Contrary to earlier practice, all DRIs except the RDAs are useful for the assessment of nutrient intakes. The RDAs are inappropriate for the assessment of the nutrient intakes of groups because the percentage of individuals with usual intakes below the RDA does not estimate the percentage of individuals with inadequate intakes. The prevalence of inadequate intakes can be estimated by comparing usual intakes in the group to the entire distribution of requirements in the same group. This approach is known as the full probability approach and was proposed by the National Research Council (1986). The EAR cut-point method, a shortcut of the full probability approach, may also be used to obtain such an estimate (Beaton, 1994; Carriquiry, 1999; IOM, 2000). Estimation of the prevalence of nutrient inadequacy in a group by determining the proportion of individuals with

---

BOX 3-1
Definitions of Dietary Reference Intakes
Used to Plan and Assess Group Intakes

Estimated Average Requirement (EAR) An EAR is the usual daily intake level that is estimated to meet the nutrient requirements of half of the healthy individuals in a life-stage and gender group.

Adequate Intake (AI) When the evidence was insufficient to determine an EAR for a nutrient, the Institute of Medicine set AI values instead. The AI is defined as a recommended average daily nutrient intake level and is based on observed or experimentally derived intake levels or approximations of the mean nutrient intake level by a group (or groups) of apparently healthy people that are assumed to be adequate (IOM, 2006b).

Tolerable Upper Intake Level (UL) A UL is the highest daily Intake level that likely poses no risk of adverse health effects. As the usual daily intake increases above the UL, the risk of adverse effects increases. The ULs for most nutrients are based on intakes from supplements as well as intake from foods and beverages.

Acceptable Macronutrient Distribution Range (AMDR) The AMDRs are defined for energy-providing macronutrients. AMDRs define the range of usual daily intakes that is associated with a reduced risk of chronic disease while providing adequate amounts of essential nutrients.

---

intakes below the RDAs would lead to overestimation of the true prevalence of nutrient inadequacy (IOM, 2000).

DRIs are defined for 12 different life-stage and gender groups. For schoolchildren, the groups are 5–8 years (both genders), males ages 9–13 years, females ages 9–13 years, males ages 14–18 years, and females ages 14–18 years.

Evaluating Adequacy for Nutrients with an EAR

The proportion of a group with usual daily intakes below the EAR is an estimate of the prevalence of nutrient inadequacy in that population group. With the exception of iron for female adolescents, the method of choice for assessment of the prevalence of nutrient inadequacy is the EAR cut-point method (IOM, 2000, 2003). The EAR cut-point method involves estimation of the proportion of individuals in a group whose usual nutrient intakes are less than the EAR. It has been shown that, under certain assumptions, the proportion with usual intakes less than the EAR is an estimate of the proportion of a group whose usual intakes do not meet the requirements (Beaton, 1994; Carriquiry, 1999; IOM, 2000). This approach was used to estimate the prevalence of inadequate intakes within each of the CACFP age groups for protein, carbohydrates, nine vitamins (A, B_6, B_{12}, C, E, thiamin, riboflavin, niacin, and folate), and three minerals (phosphorus, magnesium, and zinc).

Some of the CACFP age groups contain more than one DRI age group; for example, the age group for children 5 to 10 years contains two: DRI age groups 4–8 years and 9–13 years. The CACFP group for females (or males) ages 19–59 years contains three DRI groups: 19–30, 31–50, and 51–60 years. When mixed CACFP age groups occurred, the committee first estimated usual nutrient intake distributions and the proportion of individuals with usual intakes below the EAR using the DRI groups. The committee then computed the weighted average of the DRI group-specific prevalence of inadequacies, where the weights were given by the proportion of persons that belonged to each DRI group in the mixed CACFP group.

For female adolescents and for women ages 19–59 years, the probability approach (NRC, 1986) was used to assess iron intake, as recommended by the IOM (2000). This more complex approach accounts for both the distribution of iron requirements (which is skewed for these age-gender groups; see IOM, 2000) and the distribution of usual intakes. Moreover, the committee increased the EAR value used for females ages 11–13 years from 5.7 mg of iron per day to 7.5 mg per day, as explained in the School Meals report (IOM, 2010, pp. 65–66). *Dietary Reference Intakes: Applications in Dietary Assessment* (IOM, 2000) provides more detailed information about the EAR cut-point and probability methods.

Evaluating Adequacy for Nutrients with an AI

Groups with mean intakes at or above the AI can generally be assumed to have a low prevalence of inadequacy for the criterion of adequate nutritional status used for that nutrient. Assumptions about the inadequacy of intakes cannot be made when the mean intake is below the AI. As described by the IOM (2000), the inherent limitations of the AI affect the inferences that can be made about the prevalence of inadequacy for nutrients with an AI (IOM, 2000). Data were evaluated by comparing the estimated mean intakes with the AI. For the mixed DRI age groups, the committee proceeded as described above and computed the weighted average of the mean intakes divided by the age-appropriate AIs.

Evaluating the Risk of Excessive Intake

The proportion of a group with intakes above the UL is an estimate of the prevalence of intakes at risk of being excessive. The data from NHANES

2003–2004 do not include contributions from dietary supplements. For this reason, the committee's assessment of usual nutrient intakes relative to ULs focused primarily on intakes of sodium.

Usual intakes of saturated fat and cholesterol were compared with the recommendations in the 2005 *Dietary Guidelines for Americans* (HHS/USDA, 2005) to determine the percentage of individuals in each age group with intakes that exceeded the recommendations.

Evaluating Ranges of Energy Intake from Macronutrients

AMDRs are expressed as a percentage of the total energy intake. For example, the AMDR for fat for children ages 4 through 18 years is 25 to 35 percent of the total energy intake. For these nutrients, the proportion of an age group that fell within defined AMDRs, as well as proportions with usual intakes that either exceeded or fell below the AMDRs, was examined.

SUMMARY

NHANES 2003–2004, plus the MPED 2.0, were the primary sources of dietary data used by the committee. The standards against which intakes were measured included AAP recommendations for those younger than 2 years, the 2005 *Dietary Guidelines for Americans* (HHS/USDA, 2005) for those 2 years and older, and the DRIs for persons across the entire age span. Mean food intakes for those ages 2 years and older were evaluated by comparison with MyPyramid food pattern recommendations for selected calorie levels. Nutrient intakes were evaluated using the IOM methodology. Results of these evaluations appear in the next two chapters.

REFERENCES

AAP (American Academy of Pediatrics). 1999. Iron fortification of infant formulas. *Pediatrics* 104(1 I):119–123.

AAP. 2001a. WIC program. *Pediatrics* 108(5):1216–1217.

AAP. 2001b. American Academy of Pediatrics: The use and misuse of fruit juice in pediatrics. *Pediatrics* 107(5):1210–1213.

AAP. 2005. Breastfeeding and the use of human milk. *Pediatrics* 115(2):496–506.

AAP. 2009. *Pediatric Nutrition Handbook*, 6th ed. Elk Grove Village, IL: AAP.

ADA (American Dietetic Association). 2004. Position of the American Dietetic Association: Dietary guidance for healthy children ages 2 to 11 years. *Journal of the American Dietetic Association* 104(4):660–677.

Ard, J. D., C. J. Coffman, P. H. Lin, and L. P. Svetkey. 2004. One-year follow-up study of blood pressure and dietary patterns in Dietary Approaches to Stop Hypertension (DASH)-Sodium participants. *American Journal of Hypertension* 17(12):1156–1162.

Appel, L. J., M. W. Brands, S. R. Daniels, N. Karanja, P. J. Elmer, and F. M. Sacks. 2006. Dietary approaches to prevent and treat hypertension: A scientific statement from the American Heart Association. *Hypertension* 47(2):296–308.

Bartali, B., S. Salvini, A. Turrini, F. Lauretani, C. R. Russo, A. M. Corsi, S. Bandinelli, A. D'Amicis, D. Palli, J. M. Guralnik, and L. Ferrucci. 2003. Age and disability affect dietary intake. *Journal of Nutrition* 133(9):2868–2873.

Basch, C. E., S. Shea, R. Arliss, I. R. Contento, J. Rips, B. Gutin, M. Irigoyen, and P. Zybert. 1990. Validation of mothers' reports of dietary intake by four to seven year-old children. *American Journal of Public Health* 80(11):1314–1317.

Beaton, G. H. 1994. Approaches to analysis of dietary data: Relationship between planned analyses and choice of methodology. *American Journal of Clinical Nutrition* 59(1 Suppl): 253S–261S.

Braam, L., A. J. Lavienja, M. C. Ocke, H. B. Bueno-De-Mesquita, and J. C. Seidell. 1998. Determinants of obesity-related underreporting of energy intake. *American Journal of Epidemiology* 147(11):1081–1086.

Bratteby, L., B. Sandhagen, H. Fan, H. Enghardt, and G. Samuelson. 1998. Total energy expenditure and physical activity as assessed by the doubly labeled water method in Swedish adolescents in whom energy intake was underestimated by 7-d diet records. *American Journal Clinical Nutrition* 67(5):905–911.

Carriquiry, A. L. 1999. Assessing the prevalence of nutrient inadequacy. *Public Health Nutrition* 2(1):23–33.

Fisher, J. O., R. K. Johnson, C. Lindquist, L. L. Birch, and M. I. Goran. 2000. Influence of body composition on the accuracy of reported energy intake in children. *Obesity Research* 8(8):597–603.

Fuller, W. A. 2009. *Sampling Statistics*. Hoboken, NJ: John Wiley & Sons.

HHS/USDA (U.S. Department of Health and Human Services/U.S. Department of Agriculture). 2005. *Dietary Guidelines for Americans*, 6th ed. Washington, DC: U.S. Government Printing Office. http://www.health.gov/DietaryGuidelines/dga2005/document/ (accessed July 23, 2008).

IOM (Institute of Medicine). 2000. *Dietary Reference Intakes: Applications in Dietary Assessment*. Washington, DC: National Academy Press.

IOM. 2002/2005. *Dietary Reference Intakes for Energy, Carbohydrate, Fiber, Fat, Fatty Acids, Cholesterol, Protein, and Amino Acids*. Washington, DC: The National Academies Press.

IOM. 2003. *Dietary Reference Intakes: Applications in Dietary Planning*. Washington, DC: The National Academies Press.

IOM. 2006a. *WIC Food Packages: Time for a Change*. Washington, DC: The National Academies Press.

IOM. 2006b. *Dietary Reference Intakes: The Essential Guide to Nutrient Requirements*. Washington, DC: The National Academies Press.

IOM. 2010. *School Meals: Building Blocks for Healthy Children*. Washington, DC: The National Academies Press.

ISU (Iowa State University). 1997. Software for Intake Distribution Estimation (PC-SIDE), Version 1.02. ISU, Ames.

Johnson, R. K., B. A. Yon, and J. H. Hankin. 2008. Dietary assessment and validation. In *Research: Successful Approaches*, 3rd ed., edited by E. R. Monsen and L. Van Horn. Chicago, IL: American Dietetic Association.

Kleinman, R. E. 2000. American Academy of Pediatrics recommendations for complementary feeding. *Pediatrics* 106(5 II):1274.

Krebs, N. F., J. E. Westcott, N. Butler, C. Robinson, M. Bell, and K. M. Hambidge. 2006. Meat as a first complementary food for breastfed infants: Feasibility and impact on zinc intake and status. *Journal of Pediatric Gastroenterology and Nutrition* 42(2):207–214.

Kretsch, M. J., A. K. H. Fong, and M. W. Green. 1999. Behavioral and body size correlates of energy intake underreporting by obese and normal-weight women. *Journal of the American Dietetic Association* 99(3):300–306.

Kuczmarski, R. J., C. L. Ogden, L. M. Grummer-Strawn, K. M. Flegal, S. S. Guo, R. Wei, Z. Mei, L. R. Curtin, A. F. Roche, and C. L. Johnson. 2000. CDC growth charts: United States. *Advance Data from Vital and Health Statistics* (314):1–28. http://www.cdc.gov/nchs/data/ad/ad314.pdf (accessed July 28, 2009).

Little, P., J. Barnett, B. Margetts, A. L. Kinmonth, J. Gabbay, R. Thompson, D. Warm, H. Warwick, and S. Wooton. 1999. The validity of dietary assessment in general practice. *Journal of Epidemiology and Community Health* 53(3):165–172.

Livingstone, M. B. E., and P. J. Robson. 2000. Measurement of dietary intake in children. *Proceedings of the Nutrition Society* 59(2):279–293.

Lytle, L. A., M. Z. Nichaman, E. Obarzanek, E. Glovsky, D. Montgomery, T. Nicklas, M. Zive, and H. Feldman. 1993. Validation of 24-hour recalls assisted by food records in third-grade children. *Journal of the American Dietetic Association* 93(12):1431–1436.

Marcoe, K., W. Juan, S. Yamini, A. Carlson, and P. Britten. 2006. Development of food group composites and nutrient profiles for the MyPyramid food guidance system. *Journal of Nutrition Education and Behavior* 38(6 Suppl):S93–S107.

Moshfegh, A. J., D. G. Rhodes, D. J. Baer, T. Murayi, J. C. Clemens, W. V. Rumpler, D. R. Paul, R. S. Sebastian, K. J. Kuczynski, L. A. Ingwersen, R. C. Staples, and L. E. Cleveland. 2008. The US Department of Agriculture Automated Multiple-Pass Method reduces bias in the collection of energy intakes. *American Journal of Clinical Nutrition* 88(2):324–332.

Nestlé Nutrition Institute. 2009. *FITS Feeding Infants and Toddlers Study: 2008 Preliminary Findings.* http://medical.gerber.com/nirf/cm2/upload/20446F1F-6EB9-4D23-9151-759BC6F598B3/2385_FITS08-PrelimFind-FINALv2-05.pdf (accessed October 4, 2010).

NHLBI (National Heart, Lung, and Blood Institute). 2010. *Your Guide to Lowering Blood Pressure: Healthy Eating.* http://www.nhlbi.nih.gov/hbp/prevent/h_eating/h_eating.htm (accessed October 11, 2010).

NRC (National Research Council). 1986. *Nutrient Adequacy: Assessment Using Food Consumption Surveys.* Washington, DC: National Academy Press.

NRC. 1989. *Recommended Dietary Allowances*, 10th ed. Washington, DC: National Academy Press.

Nusser, S. M., A. L. Carriquiry, K. W. Dodd, and W. A. Fuller. 1996. A semiparametric transformation approach to estimating usual daily intake distributions. *Journal of the American Statistical Association* 91(436):1440–1449.

Sacks, F. M., L. P. Svetkey, W. M. Vollmer, L. J. Appel, G. A. Bray, D. Harsha, E. Obarzanek, P. R. Conlin, E. R. Miller III, D. G. Simons-Morton, N. Karanja, P. H. Lin, M. Aickin, M. M. Most-Windhauser, T. J. Moore, M. A. Proschan, and J. A. Cutler. 2001. Effects on blood pressure of reduced dietary sodium and the Dietary Approaches to Stop Hypertension (DASH) diet. *New England Journal of Medicine* 344(1):3–10.

Scagliusi, F. B., V. O. Polacow, G. G. Artioli, F. B. Benatti, and A. H. Lancha, Jr. 2003. Selective underreporting of energy intake in women: Magnitude, determinants, and effect of training. *Journal of the American Dietetic Association* 103(10):1306–1313.

Sharkey, J. R. 2008. Diet and health outcomes in vulnerable populations. *Annals of the New York Academy of Sciences* 1136:210–217.

Subar, A. F., V. Kipnis, R. P. Troiano, D. Midthune, D. A. Schoeller, S. Bingham, C. O. Sharbaugh, J. Trabulsi, S. Runswick, R. Ballard-Barbash, J. Sunshine, and A. Schatzkin. 2003. Using intake biomarkers to evaluate the extent of dietary misreporting in a large sample of adults: The OPEN study. *American Journal of Epidemiology* 158(1):1–13.

USDA (U.S. Department of Agriculture). 2009. *Inside the Pyramid.* http://www.mypyramid.gov/pyramid/index.html (accessed October 19, 2010).

USDA/ARS (U.S. Department of Agriculture/Agricultural Research Service). 2000. *1994–1996 Continuing Survey of Food Intakes by Individuals (CSFII 1994–1996) and 1998 Supplemental Children's Survey (CSFII 1998).* Beltsville, MD: ARS.

USDA/ARS. 2004. *What We Eat in America, NHANES 2001–2002*: Documentation and data files. Washington, DC: USDA/ARS. http://www.ars.usda.gov/main/site_main.htm?modecode= 12-35-50-00 (accessed August 9, 2010).

USDA/ARS. 2010a. *What We Eat in America, NHANES 2007–2008*. http://www.ars.usda. gov/Services/docs.htm?docid=18349 (accessed October 5, 2010).

USDA/ARS. 2010b. *What We Eat in America, NHANES 2003–2004*. http://www.ars.usda. gov/Services/docs.htm?docid=18349 (accessed October 21, 2010).

WHO (World Health Organization). 2002. *The Optimal Duration of Exclusive Breastfeeding: Report of an Expert Consultation*. Geneva, Switzerland: WHO. http://www.who. int/nutrition/publications/optimal_duration_of_exc_bfeeding_report_eng.pdf (accessed July 9, 2010).

WHO. 2003. *Complementary Feeding: Report of the Global Consultation, and Summary of Guiding Principles for Complementary Feeding of the Breastfed Child*. Geneva, Switzerland: WHO. http://whqlibdoc.who.int/publications/2002/924154614X.pdf (accessed July 9, 2010).

Ziegler, P., R. Briefel, N. Clusen, and B. Devaney. 2006. Feeding Infants and Toddlers Study (FITS): Development of the FITS survey in comparison to other dietary survey methods. *Journal of the American Dietetic Association* 106(1 Suppl):S12–S27.

4

Nutritional Considerations
for Infants and Children

This chapter presents the committee's findings regarding food and nutrient intakes by infants and children. Food intakes by infants and children are compared to findings about current dietary guidance, and nutrient intakes are considered in relation to Dietary Reference Intakes (DRIs). The chapter includes special nutritional considerations relating to weight status, bone health, and iron status. Key foods and nutrients that need to be encouraged or are of concern are identified.

To examine food and nutrient intakes and identify concerns, the committee used the data sets, other source materials, and methods that are described in Chapter 3. In many cases, the committee referred to the analyses conducted for the reports *WIC Food Packages: Time for a Change* (IOM, 2006) and *School Meals: Building Blocks for Healthy Children* (IOM, 2010), because those analyses cover the age groups as those served in the Child and Adult Care Food Program (CACFP).

FOOD INTAKES

Infants and Children Younger Than 2 Years of Age

Infants and children younger than 2 years of age are considered together because dietary guidance for this group relies on recommendations of the American Academy of Pediatrics (AAP, 2009). The *Dietary Guidelines for Americans* does not apply to persons younger than 2 years of age. The age groups of interest are 0–5 months, 6–11 months, and 1 year.

Zero Through 5 Months of Age

Although exclusive breastfeeding is recommended for infants up to 6 months of age (AAP, 2009), breastfeeding proportions in the United States range from 74 percent shortly after birth to 14 percent exclusively breastfeeding at 6 months (CDC, 2010). Breastfeeding prevalence is lower among women in low-income groups than for the general population: 71 percent for those at 100–184 percent of the poverty threshold compared to 78 percent for those at 185–349 percent of poverty (CDC, 2010). The first Feeding Infants and Toddlers Study (FITS), a comprehensive assessment of food and nutrient intakes of infants and toddlers, found that almost 30 percent of infants were fed complementary foods before the age of 4 months, when infants should be consuming only breast milk or formula (Briefel et al., 2004). The AAP, in its most recent recommendations, advises that the introduction of complementary foods be delayed until after 6 months of age (AAP, 2009) (also see Chapter 3, Table 3-1).

Six Months Through 1 Year of Age

A study of participants in the Supplemental Nutrition Program for Women, Infants, and Children (WIC) (USDA/FCS, 1997) found, like the FITS study (Fox et al., 2004), that many 6–11-month-old infants had been introduced to foods earlier than recommended. Almost 25 percent of infants ages 9 through 11 months were fed cow's milk (Briefel et al., 2004; USDA/FCS, 1997), which AAP (2009) recommends delaying until 1 year of age. Fruit juice intake exceeded AAP recommendations for about 60 percent of the children ages 1–2 years old in FITS (Skinner et al., 2004). Nonjuice fruit and vegetable consumption was low, with approximately 30 percent of infants and toddlers consuming no fruits or vegetables (Fox et al., 2004). The most common vegetable consumed by toddlers 15 months and older was fried potatoes (Fox et al., 2004).

Fox et al. (2006) reported that juice was second only to milk in the amount of energy contributed to the diets of children age 1 year. Among the other foods also reported to contribute significant percentages of the energy intake of children age 1 year were several that are high in solid fat and/or added sugars. These include sweetened beverages (4.7 percent of energy), cookies (3.2 percent), cakes and pies (1.7 percent), and chips and other salty snacks (1.3 percent), among others. Also, notably, more than 60 percent of 1-year-old children enrolled in WIC had usual sodium intakes above the Tolerable Upper Intake Level (UL) (IOM, 2006).

Children Ages 2 Through 18 Years

For each of the MyPyramid food groups, Table 4-1 shows the recommended amounts of food in the MyPyramid patterns and the usual mean intakes at five comparable calorie/age group levels. The basis for comparing food intake data with MyPyramid patterns and for using these age and calorie levels is presented in Chapter 3. Table 4-1 also includes data on the intake of oils and calories from discretionary solid fats and added sugars.

Summary of Food Intake Findings Compared with MyPyramid Amounts

Analysis of the National Health and Nutrition Examination Survey (NHANES 2003–2004) indicates that the intake of dark green vegetables, orange vegetables, and legumes was very low, which is consistent with findings in previous Institute of Medicine reports (IOM, 2006, 2010). Total vegetable intake was low as well, and a substantial portion of the vegetables were in the form of fried potatoes or chips (USDA/FNS, 2008, Table C-22). Compared with vegetable intake, total fruit intake was somewhat closer to the MyPyramid recommendation. However, especially for the younger children, juice accounted for much of the fruit. The consumption of whole grains was very low; however, for most groups, mean total grain intake (nearly all of which was refined grain) was higher than the amount specified in the MyPyramid patterns. The *Dietary Guidelines* (HHS/USDA, 2005) specifically encourages the intake of a variety of vegetables and three or more ounce-equivalents (or at least half of the grains consumed) as whole grains each day. Total mean milk group intake by the youngest age group exceeded the MyPyramid amount shown in Table 4-1. Although the recommended amount of milk increases from 2 to 3 cups at age 9 years, the mean amount consumed actually decreases with age. Mean intakes of meat and beans were about 60 to 80 percent of MyPyramid amounts.

Intakes of Solid Fats and Added Sugars

As shown in Table 4-1, children's mean daily intakes of calories from solid fats and added sugars are very high. The 2010 Dietary Guidelines Advisory Committee (USDA/HHS, 2010) emphasizes the importance of reducing intakes of these ingredients in the diet of all Americans, especially children. Estimates from the U.S. Department of Agriculture (USDA) suggest that, for school-age children, the highest contributors of solid fat include sandwiches such as burgers (15 percent), fried potatoes, and pizza with meat, which contributed about 6 percent each (USDA/FNS, 2008,

TABLE 4-1 Comparison of MyPyramid Food Group Patterns with Mean Daily Amounts of MyPyramid Food Groups Consumed by Children, by Age Group

Food Group or Component[a]	2–4 Years		5–13 Years			14–18 Years	
	1,300 kcal Pattern[b]	Mean Intake 2–4 Years	1,900 kcal Pattern[c]	Mean Intake 5–10 Years[d]	Mean Intake 11–13 Years[d]	2,400 kcal Pattern	Mean Intake 14–18 Years[d]
Total fruit (cup eq)	1.25	1.54	1.75	1.09	0.96	2	0.94
Total vegetables (cup eq)	1.5	0.89	2.5	1.11	1.15	3	1.36
Dark green	0.21[e]	0.03	0.43[e]	0.03	0.04	0.43[e]	0.04
Orange	0.14[e]	0.06	0.29[e]	0.04	0.04	0.29[e]	0.04
Dry beans/peas	0.14[e]	0.06	0.43[e]	0.08	0.09	0.43[e]	0.10
Starchy	0.36[e]	0.35	0.43[e]	0.42	0.39	0.86[e]	0.45
Other	0.64[e]	0.39	0.93[e]	0.54	0.59	1[e]	0.73
Total grains (oz eq)	4.5	4.91	6	6.79	7.25	8	7.57
Whole grains (oz eq)	2.25	0.49	3	0.59	0.48	4	0.42
Total meat and beans (oz eq)[f]	3.5	2.97	5.25	3.16	3.97	6.5	4.36
Total milk group (8 fl oz eq)[g]	2	2.29	3	2.46	2.17	3	2.18
Vegetable oils (g)[b]	17	12	26	15	17	31	20
SoFAS (kcal)	171	567[i]	231	778[i]	781[i]	362	897[i]

NOTES: The MyPyramid food intake pattern used is from the *Dietary Guidelines for Americans* (HHS/USDA, 2005). Eq = equivalent; fl = fluid; g = gram; kcal = calories; oz = ounce; SoFAS = solid fats and added sugars.

[a]See Appendix Table H-1 for a list of foods in the MyPyramid food groups and subgroups.

[b]1,300-calorie pattern based on an average of the 1,200- and 1,400-calorie patterns.

[c]1,900-calorie pattern based on an average of the 1,800- and 2,000-calorie patterns.

[d]Average of male and female intake data.

[e]Daily amounts based on the MyPyramid recommendations expressed as cup equivalents per week.

[f]The MyPyramid meat and beans group includes meat, poultry, fish, eggs, dry beans and peas, and nuts and seeds (http://www.mypyramid.gov/pyramid/meat.html).

[g]The MyPyramid milk group includes fluid milk; hard, soft, and processed cheese; yogurt; and milk-based desserts (http://www.mypyramid.gov/pyramid/milk.html). The intake data represent mean intake of fluid milk, cheese, and yogurt. *Dietary Guidelines* advises "3 cups per day of fat-free or low-fat milk or equivalent milk products" for children ages 9 years and older; 2 cups per day for younger children (see HHS/USDA, 2005, p. viii).

[h]5 g = 1 teaspoon.

[i]Estimated on the basis of the number of grams (g) of discretionary solid fat and the number of teaspoons (tsp) of added sugars, as follows: (fat g × 9 calories/g) + (tsp × 4.2 g/tsp × 4 calories/g).

SOURCES: Mean intake data from NHANES 2003–2004; MyPyramid patterns from Britten et al., 2006.

TABLE 4-2 Estimated Prevalence of Inadequacy of Selected Micronutrients and Protein Using Usual Intakes in Infants

	Estimated Prevalence of Inadequacy (%)	
Nutrient	WIC Infants, Nonbreastfed, 6–11 Months ($n = 275$)	Breastfed Infants, 6–11 Months[a] ($n = 143$)
Iron	1.7	39.5
Zinc	0.3	60.3
Protein	0.6	—[a]

NOTES: n = sample size.

[a]Because of the lack of data on the quantity of breast milk consumed by breast-fed infants 6–11 months of age, protein adequacy could not be assessed. Iron and zinc adequacy could be estimated because breast milk consumed by breastfed infants has little iron and zinc content. SOURCES: Adapted from IOM, 2006, Table 2-1. Intake data are from 1994–1996 and 1998 *Continuing Survey of Food Intake by Individuals* (USDA/ARS, 2000); data set does not include intake from dietary supplements (e.g., multivitamin and mineral preparations). Intake distributions were calculated using PC-SIDE (ISU, 1997). Estimated Average Requirements used in the analysis were from the Dietary Reference Intake reports (IOM, 2001, 2002/2005).

Table C-29). By far the largest contributors to children's intake of added sugars (45 percent of the total amount) are regular soda and noncarbonated sweetened drinks (USDA/FNS, 2008, Table C-30).

NUTRIENT INTAKES

Infants

Data on nutrient intakes by infants, especially very young and/or breastfed infants are limited. Reporting on findings from the first FITS, which included both formula-fed and breastfed infants, Briefel and colleagues (2006) show that Hispanic and non-Hispanic infants ages 4 and 5 months had usual intakes that were all well above the respective Adequate Intakes (AIs) of the 11 micronutrients that were studied.[1] For infants ages 6–11 months, mean intakes exceeded the AI for 9 micronutrients.[2]

Table 4-2, adapted from *WIC Food Packages* (IOM, 2006), which used data from the 1990s, shows that the prevalence of inadequate iron and zinc intakes were quite high among breastfed compared to formula-fed infants ages 6–11 months. Iron and zinc are the only micronutrients for

---

[1]Vitamins A, C, D, E, folate, and B_{12}; calcium, iron, phosphorus, potassium, and zinc.

[2]Vitamins A, C, D, E, folate, and B_{12}; calcium, phosphorus, and potassium. Iron and zinc are not included because an Estimated Average Requirement (EAR) rather than an AI has been set for infants ages 6–11 months.

which EARs have been set for older infants. The prevalence of inadequacy of protein intake was very low for nonbreastfed infants, ages 6–11 months, and is assumed to be very low for breastfed infants.

Children and Adolescents

Estimates of Energy Intake

In several recent reports (IOM, 2006, 2010; Ziegler et al., 2006), major discrepancies were found between the mean energy intake that was estimated using nationally representative data and the mean Estimated Energy Requirement (EER) that was calculated as described in Chapter 3. For example, reported usual energy intakes exceeded the mean EER by about 400 calories for the younger school-age children, and the energy intakes were lower than the EER for adolescents ages 14–18 years (IOM, 2010). Possible reasons for these discrepancies in estimated energy intake and expenditure include (1) over-reporting of total food intake and underestimation of physical activity level for younger children and (2) under-reporting of total food intake and overestimation of physical activity level by the adolescents. These discrepancies limited the committee's ability to draw conclusions about the adequacy of energy intake using survey data, but nationally representative data on the prevalence of childhood overweight and obesity provide strong reason for concern about excessive calorie intake (see "Weight Status" under "Special Nutritional Considerations" later in this chapter).

Estimates of Nutrient Inadequacy

Using methods described in Chapter 3, the committee estimated the prevalence of inadequacy of protein and selected vitamins and minerals among children ages 1–18 years. The results are presented by age group in Table 4-3.

In agreement with findings reported in earlier IOM publications (IOM, 2006, 2010), a high prevalence of inadequacy was found for vitamins A, C, and E; phosphorus; and, for adolescents, magnesium (bold values in Table 4-3). In general, the prevalence of inadequacy increased with age and was higher for females than for males. Notably, females ages 14–18 years had a high prevalence of inadequacy for 10 of the 14 nutrients examined. The findings for this group of females are consistent with their low reported mean energy intakes.

TABLE 4-3 Estimated Prevalence of Inadequacy of Protein and Selected Vitamins and Minerals Among Children Based on Usual Nutrient Intakes from NHANES[a]

| | | | Estimated Prevalence of Inadequate Usual Intakes (%) | | | | | |
| | | | 5–10 Years | | 11–13 Years | | 14–18 Years | |
	1 Year	2–4 Years	Males	Females	Males	Females	Males	Females
Protein	0	0	0.6	**3.3**	**1.8**	**6**	**6**	**12**
Vitamin A	1.6	1.8	**11**	**13**	**29**	**32**	**62**	**56**
Vitamin C	0.2	1.2	**6**	**5**	**9**	**8**	**39**	**42**
Vitamin E	**82**	**82**	**86**	**88**	**88**	**95**	**94**	**100**
Thiamin	0	0	0	0	0.1	0	4.9	0
Riboflavin	0	0	0	0.2	0.1	0.5	2.2	1.0
Niacin	0.3	0.2	0.1	0.1	0.2	0.2	0.4	0.2
Vitamin B$_6$	0	0	0.2	0.4	0.6	1.1	**5**	**10**
Folate	0.2	0.1	0.2	0.1	0.6	0.3	**8**	**14**
Vitamin B$_{12}$	0	0	0	0.1	0.1	0.3	0.3	2.4
Phosphorus	0.2	0.1	1.0	**13**	**12**	**39**	**14**	**37**
Magnesium	0.1	0.2	**7**	**15**	**20**	**45**	**79**	**95**
Iron	1.5	0.7	0.2	0.2	0	**7**[b]	1.2	**9**
Zinc	0.1	0.1	0.6	2.9	**1.8**	**9**	**5**	**11**

NOTES: Bold font indicates values with a prevalence of inadequacy greater than 5 percent. Includes pregnant and lactating women.

[a]All nutrients in this table have an Estimated Average Requirement (EAR).

[b]Methods used to calculate iron values for females 11–13 years old are described in Chapter 3.

SOURCES: Intake data from NHANES 2003–2004. The EARs used in the analysis were from the Dietary Reference Intake reports (IOM, 1997, 1998, 2000, 2001, 2002/2005).

Estimates for Nutrients with an Adequate Intake Value

The mean and median intakes for five nutrients (calcium, potassium, fiber, linoleic acid, and α-linolenic acid) were identified by age group and are shown in relation to the AI (see Table 4-4). Sodium is not included in Table 4-4 because the concern is for excessive rather than inadequate sodium intake. Data on vitamin D intakes were not available for the age groups used in this study. However, the recent *What We Eat in America* survey (USDA/ARS, 2009) includes estimates of vitamin D intakes (for different age groups) and indicates low intakes, especially for adolescent females.

Table 4-4 shows that mean intakes of potassium and fiber were below the AI for all five age groups and that mean intake of calcium was below the AI for the older two age groups and for the 5–10-year-old girls (bold values in Table 4-4). The mean intakes of linoleic and α-linolenic acids were above the AI for all five age groups. It is important to note a concurrent IOM study is reviewing the DRIs for vitamin D and calcium; and

TABLE 4-4 Comparison of Mean and Median Nutrient Intakes from NHANES with the Adequate Intake (AI), by Age Group and Gender

	1 Year	2–4 Years	5–10 Years Males	5–10 Years Females	11–13 Years Males	11–13 Years Females	14–18 Years Males	14–18 Years Females
Calcium (mg/d)								
AI	500	600	967	967	1,300	1,300	1,300	1,300
Mean intake	989	999	1,034	971	**1,099**	**907**	**1,202**	**852**
Median intake	954	966	995	**939**	**1,070**	**876**	**1,140**	**815**
Potassium (mg/d)								
AI	3,000	3,267	4,033	4,033	4,500	4,500	4,700	4,700
Mean intake	**2,177**	**2,184**	**2,293**	**2,166**	**2,432**	**2,097**	**2,848**	**2,099**
Median intake	**2,103**	**2,114**	**2,229**	**2,125**	**2,370**	**2,057**	**2,755**	**2,040**
Fiber (g/d)								
AI	19.0	21.0	27.0	25.3	31.0	26.0	38.0	26.0
Mean intake	**9.5**	**10.1**	**12.6**	**12.0**	**14.3**	**12.4**	**15.4**	**12.0**
Median intake	**9.1**	**9.8**	**12.2**	**11.7**	**13.8**	**12.1**	**14.6**	**11.5**
Linoleic acid (g/d)								
AI	7.0	8.0	10.7	10.0	12.0	10.0	16.0	11.0
Mean intake	8.2	9.1	12.9	12.0	15.4	13.1	16.5	14.1
Median intake	7.8	8.7	12.2	11.6	14.9	12.7	15.5	13.4
α-Linolenic acid (g/d)								
AI	0.7	0.8	1.0	0.9	1.2	1.0	1.6	1.1
Mean intake	0.9	1.0	1.2	1.2	1.4	1.2	1.6	1.3
Median intake	0.9	0.9	1.2	1.1	1.3	1.2	**1.5**	1.3

NOTES: AI = Adequate Intake; g/d = grams per day; mg/d = milligrams per day; NHANES = National Health and Nutrition Examination Survey. Bold font indicates mean and median intake values lower than the AI.
SOURCES: Intake data from NHANES 2003–2004. The AIs used in the analysis were from the DRI reports (IOM, 1997, 2002/2005, 2005). AIs shown for the 2–4-year-old and 5–10-year-old age groups are weighted averages of the AIs for two DRI age groups.

the recommendations from this study may have implications for CACFP participants' requirements of these nutrients.

Usual Intakes of Macronutrients

Intakes of protein and total carbohydrate generally were within the respective Acceptable Macronutrient Distribution Range (AMDR) (IOM, 2006, 2010). For total fat intakes, about 18 percent of children ages 2–4 years who participated in WIC had intakes *below* the lower bound of the AMDR (IOM, 2006), whereas nearly the same percentage of school-age children had total fat intakes that were *above* the upper bound (35 percent) of the AMDR (IOM, 2010). Notably, however, over 3 percent of females ages 14–18 years had low reported fat intakes (USDA/FNS, 2008).

Excessive Intake Levels

In general, the risk of excessive nutrient intakes was low for children. Some notable exceptions follow:

- Intakes of sodium were clearly excessive for all children ages 2 years and older. Analysis of data from NHANES 2003–2004 shows that more than 80 percent of children ages 1 through 4 years and 83 to 97 percent of school-age children had usual sodium intakes above the UL. This may be an underestimate in that the data sets used for these analyses did not include dietary sodium added in the form of table salt.
- Approximately 58 percent of WIC children ages 2–4 years had usual zinc intakes above the UL, and about 16 percent of WIC children also had usual intakes of preformed vitamin A above the UL (IOM, 2006). For school-age children, intakes at the 95th percentile of the distribution were well below the ULs for all nutrients with a UL except zinc (IOM, 2010). The zinc intakes that exceeded the UL were observed primarily among children ages 6–8 years. These estimates of children with zinc intakes above the UL are likely low because the data set for these analyses did not include intake from dietary supplements.
- As found in other reports (IOM, 2006, 2010; USDA/HHS, 2010), analysis of NHANES 2003–2004 data revealed that high percentages (77 to 88 percent) of children ages 3 years and older had saturated fat intakes above the maximum of 10 percent of total food energy advised in the *Dietary Guidelines for Americans* (HHS/USDA, 2005). The 2010 Dietary Guidelines Advisory Committee (USDA/HHS, 2010) recommended moving toward a goal of no more than 7 percent of total food energy from saturated fat.
- The 2005 *Dietary Guidelines* (HHS/USDA, 2005) recommends 300 mg of cholesterol as the maximum daily intake (for all persons who are at least 2 years of age). Cholesterol intakes were fairly consistent with the recommendation, but the prevalence of NHANES 2003–2004 intakes in excess of 300 mg per day increased with increasing energy intake. The prevalence of excessive intake was highest among adolescent males (nearly 16 percent for males ages 11–13 years and nearly 47 percent for males ages 14–18 years). The preliminary report from the 2010 Dietary Guidelines Advisory Committee (USDA/HHS, 2010) recommends moving toward a goal of no more than 200 mg of cholesterol per day. Many children have intakes that would exceed this level.

SPECIAL NUTRITIONAL CONSIDERATIONS

The food- and nutrient-related reference standards that the committee used for examining diet—namely, the American Academy of Pediatrics (AAP) (2009) feeding recommendations for infants and children younger than 2 years (see Chapter 3, Table 3-1), the 2005 *Dietary Guidelines* (including the MyPyramid patterns, which interpret the guidelines into meals and snacks), and the DRIs—allow a nearly complete examination of foods and nutrients that need to be encouraged or are of concern. It is essential, however, to consider several additional nutrition and health topics: weight status and selected related conditions, and bone health, as discussed below.

Weight Status

The *Dietary Guidelines* (HHS/USDA, 2005) place a strong emphasis on healthy weight, and the 2010 Dietary Guidelines Advisory Committee (USDA/HHS, 2010), in its preliminary report, emphasizes healthy weight even more strongly. The current guidelines encourage eating and physical activity practices that help reduce the risk of becoming overweight or obese, as defined below. Among the many reasons to emphasize healthy body weight in childhood are the strong associations between obesity and cardiovascular disease risk, hypertension, dyslipidemias (abnormal blood lipid values), and type 2 diabetes—conditions that may begin in childhood and continue into adulthood.

Assessment of Weight Status

The examination of weight status requires the use of stature (length in infants and toddlers, height for children over 2 or 3 years of age) and weight measurements. For infants and toddlers, the committee used the National Center for Health Statistics definition for excess weight, namely, the gender-specific 2000 Centers for Disease Control and Prevention (CDC) weight-for-length growth charts (NCHS, 2007) to define obesity. For children and adolescents ages 2–18 years, the committee used body mass index (BMI) to categorize weight status. The BMI is calculated by dividing the weight in kilograms by the height in meters squared (kg/m^2). This index is a good proxy for body fatness at the population level. The committee used the age- and gender-specific reference data for BMI for children published by the CDC (Kuczmarski et al., 2000) as the standard and adopted the CDC terms *obese* for children and adolescents with a BMI over the 95th percentile and *overweight* for those with a BMI between the 85th and 95th percentiles (CDC, 2009).

Obesity is prevalent among U.S. children from infancy through adoles-

TABLE 4-5 Prevalence of Overweight and Obesity Among U.S. Children, by Age, 2007–2008

| Age Group (in years, both genders) | Percentage of Children (95% CI) with High BMI Determined from CDC Growth Charts | | |
	≥ 85th Percentile	≥ 95th Percentile	≥ 97th Percentile
2–5	21.2 (17.3–25.1)	10.4 (7.6–13.1)	6.9 (4.8–9.0)
6–11	35.5 (32.4–38.7)	19.6 (17.1–22.2)	14.5 (12.2–16.8)
12–19	34.2 (30.5–37.8)	18.1 (14.5–21.7)	12.5 (9.9–15.0)

NOTES: Data from the National Health and Nutrition Examination Survey. Pregnant adolescents were excluded. Values for BMIs were rounded to one decimal place. BMI = body mass index; CDC = Centers for Disease Control and Prevention; CI = confidence interval.
SOURCE: Derived from Ogden et al., 2010.

cence. Data from the 2007–2008 NHANES reveal that 9.5 percent of all U.S. children from birth to 2 years of age had high weight for length (>95th percentile) (Ogden et al., 2010). Table 4-5 shows that, during the same period, the prevalence of overweight and of obesity was high for all children ages 2 years and older and was highest in the group ages 6–11 years.

In another analysis of the NHANES 2007–2008 data, Koebnick et al. (2010) found that, of all the ethnic-racial groups considered, non-Hispanic black adolescent children had the highest prevalence of BMI (≥ 85th percentile; 44.5 percent), and Hispanic boys had significantly higher odds of being overweight or obese compared with non-Hispanic white boys (odds ratio [OR] = 1.65 [95% confidence interval (CI): 1.14–2.38]). Non-Hispanic black girls were significantly more likely to have high BMI compared with non-Hispanic white girls (OR for > 85th percentile = 1.58 [95% CI: 0.36–0.65]). Extreme obesity, defined by Koebnick and colleagues as a BMI-for-age ≥ 1.2 times the 95th percentile by the CDC, was observed in 7.3 percent of boys and 5.5 percent of girls. The prevalence of extreme obesity varied among ethnic-racial and age groups, with the highest prevalence in Hispanic boys (as high as 11.2 percent) and African-American girls (up to 11.9 percent).

Data covering the four decades from 1963 to 2005 show that the proportion of obese children ages 2 to 19 years increased substantially (see Figure 4-1). An examination of NHANES data across the period 1999–2008 (Figure 4-2), however, demonstrates that the only statistically significant trend indicating an increased prevalence of obesity occurred at BMIs of ≥ 97th percentile for boys ages 6 through 19 years (data not shown). Even if the prevalence of obesity is no longer rising among children, the high prevalence remains of great concern to the health of the nation's children.

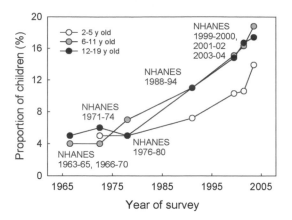

FIGURE 4-1 Prevalence of obesity (≥ 95th percentile) in boys and girls ages 2 to 19 years, 1963–2006.
SOURCE: Derived from Ogden et al., 2006, 2008.

Reasons for Concerns About Obese Weight Status in Childhood

The committee recognizes limitations in the use of BMI as a measure of pediatric obesity (see, e.g., Ebbeling and Ludwig, 2008); however, a number of studies provide evidence that childhood obesity, defined by BMI ≥ 95th percentile, is associated with certain chronic diseases and conditions. These diseases include, for example, type 2 diabetes (Messiah et al., 2008; Weiss and Caprio, 2005), hypertension (high blood pressure) (Jago et al., 2006),

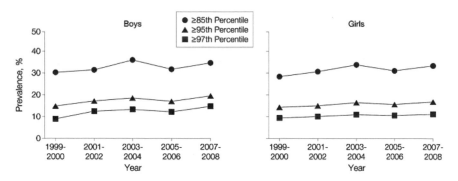

FIGURE 4-2 Prevalence of high BMI-for-age in boys and girls ages 6 through 19 years (all races), data from the 1999–2008 NHANES.
SOURCE: Ogden et al., 2010. Reprinted with permission from the *Journal of the American Medical Association*. January 2010. 303(3): 247. Copyright © (2010) American Medical Association. All rights reserved.

and metabolic syndrome (De Ferranti et al., 2006) in the short term, and both diabetes and cardiovascular disease over the long term (Baker et al., 2007). Obesity and the associated adverse effects tend to persist: children who are overweight are at increased risk of becoming overweight as adults, and overweight and obesity in adulthood increases chronic disease risk (Ferraro et al., 2003). Earlier IOM reports (IOM, 2007, 2010) on childhood obesity speak to hypertension, type 2 diabetes, metabolic syndrome, cardiovascular disease, and other conditions that are associated with obesity in more detail.

Bone Health

Nutrition and physical activity throughout life are important to bone health, but these factors are especially important during the years of bone growth and calcium accretion. About 40 percent of total skeletal bone mass is acquired within a window of 3–5 years during adolescence, when gonadal steroids and growth hormone secretion are maximal (Weaver and Heaney, 2005). Recent estimates of average calcium accretion suggest that 9–18-year-old boys and girls acquire from 92 to 210 mg of calcium per day (Vatanparast et al., 2010) and can reach peak bone calcium accretion levels ranging from 260 to 400 mg per day (Abrams et al., 2000; Bailey et al., 2000). This period of bone accretion determines adult bone mass, which may be a significant predictor of fracture risk later in life. Meals and snacks provided by the CACFP play an important role in helping children and adults consume an adequate amount of both calcium and vitamin D for bone health.

Foods and Nutrients to Be Encouraged or Limited

Infants and 1-Year-Old Children

Upon reviewing the data concerning the food and nutrient intake and weight status of children from birth through the first year, the committee determined that, in CACFP, priority should be given to promoting breastfeeding and to limiting fruit juice and foods high in solid fats, added sugars, and sodium.

Children Ages 2 Years and Older

Overall, the data on children ages 2 years and older indicate that dietary changes to improve consistency with the *Dietary Guidelines* and to improve nutrient intake would feature increased intake of a variety of vegetables, whole fruits, and whole grains; increased emphasis on low-fat or fat-free milk products; increased emphasis on very lean meats and/or beans;

and decreased intake of foods high in solid fats, added sugars, and sodium. Especially for females ages 14–18 years, the meals and snacks need to be rich in nutrients but moderate in energy content.

REFERENCES

AAP (American Academy of Pediatrics). 2009. *Pediatric Nutrition Handbook*, 6th ed. Elk Grove Village, IL: AAP.

Abrams, S. A., K. C. Copeland, et al. 2000. Calcium absorption, bone mass accumulation, and kinetics increase during early pubertal development in girls. *Journal of Clinical Endocrinology and Metabolism* 85(5):1805–1809.

Bailey, D. A., A. D. Martin, H. A. McKay, S. Whiting, and R. Mirwald. 2000. Calcium accretion in girls and boys during puberty: A longitudinal analysis. *Journal of Bone and Mineral Research* 15(11):2245–2250.

Baker, J. L., L. W. Olsen, and T. I. A. Sørensen. 2007. Childhood body-mass index and the risk of coronary heart disease in adulthood. *New England Journal of Medicine* 357(23):2329–2337.

Briefel, R. R., K. Reidy, V. Karwe, and B. Devaney. 2004. Feeding Infants and Toddlers Study: Improvements needed in meeting infant feeding recommendations. *Journal of the American Dietetic Association* 104(Suppl 1):S31–S37.

Briefel, R., P. Ziegler, T. Novak, and M. Ponza. 2006. Feeding Infants and Toddlers Study: Characteristics and usual nutrient intake of Hispanic and non-Hispanic infants and toddlers. *Journal of the American Dietetic Association* 106 (1 Suppl 1):S84–S95.

Britten, P., K. Marcoe, S. Yamini, and C. Davis. 2006. Development of Food Intake Patterns for the MyPyramid Food Guidance System. *Journal of Nutrition Education and Behavior* 38(6 Suppl.):S78–S92.

CDC (Centers for Disease Control and Prevention). 2009. *Defining Childhood Overweight and Obesity*. http://www.cdc.gov/obesity/childhood/defining.html (accessed July 10, 2009).

CDC. 2010. *National Immunization Survey, Provisional Data, 2006 births*. http://www.cdc.gov/breastfeeding/data/NIS_data/index.htm (accessed July 1, 2010).

De Ferranti, S. D., K. Gauvreau, D. S. Ludwig, J. W. Newburger, and N. Rifai. 2006. Inflammation and changes in metabolic syndrome abnormalities in US adolescents: Findings from the 1988–1994 and 1999–2000 National Health and Nutrition Examination Surveys. *Clinical Chemistry* 52(7):1325–1330.

Ebbeling, C. B., and D. S. Ludwig. 2008. Tracking pediatric obesity: An index of uncertainty? *Journal of the American Medical Association* 299(20):2442–2443.

Ferraro, K. F., R. J. Thorpe Jr, and J. A. Wilkinson. 2003. The life course of severe obesity: Does childhood overweight matter? *Journals of Gerontology, Series B: Psychological Sciences and Social Sciences* 58(2):S110–S119.

Fox, M. K., S. Pac, B. Devaney, and L. Jankowski. 2004. Feeding Infants and Toddlers study: What foods are infants and toddlers eating? *Journal of the American Dietetic Association* 104(Suppl 1):S22–S30.

Fox, M. K., K. Reidy, T. Novak, and P. Ziegler. 2006. Sources of energy and nutrients in the diets of infants and toddlers. *Journal of the American Dietetic Association* 106 (1 Suppl):S28–S42.

HHS/USDA (U.S. Department of Health and Human Services/U.S. Department of Agriculture). 2005. *Dietary Guidelines for Americans*, 6th ed. Washington, DC: U.S. Government Printing Office. http://www.health.gov/DietaryGuidelines/dga2005/document/ (accessed July 23, 2008).

IOM (Institute of Medicine). 1997. *Dietary Reference Intakes for Calcium, Phosphorus, Magnesium, Vitamin D, and Fluoride.* Washington, DC: National Academy Press.

IOM. 1998. *Dietary Reference Intakes for Thiamin, Riboflavin, Niacin, Vitamin B6, Folate, Vitamin B12, Pantothenic Acid, Biotin, and Choline.* Washington, DC: National Academy Press.

IOM. 2000. *Dietary Reference Intakes for Vitamin C, Vitamin E, Selenium, and Carotenoids.* Washington, DC: National Academy Press.

IOM. 2001. *Dietary Reference Intakes for Vitamin A, Vitamin K, Arsenic, Boron, Chromium, Copper, Iodine, Iron, Manganese, Molybdenum, Nickel, Silicon, Vanadium, and Zinc.* Washington, DC: National Academy Press.

IOM. 2002/2005. *Dietary Reference Intakes for Energy, Carbohydrate, Fiber, Fat, Fatty Acids, Cholesterol, Protein, and Amino Acids.* Washington, DC: The National Academies Press.

IOM. 2005. *Dietary Reference Intakes for Water, Potassium, Sodium, Chloride, and Sulfate.* Washington, DC: The National Academies Press.

IOM. 2006. *WIC Food Packages: Time for a Change.* Washington, DC: The National Academies Press.

IOM. 2007. *Nutrition Standards for Foods in Schools: Leading the Way Toward Healthier Youth.* Washington, DC: The National Academies Press.

IOM. 2010. *School Meals: Building Blocks for Healthy Children.* Washington, DC: The National Academies Press.

ISU (Iowa State University). 1997. *Software for Intake Distribution Estimation (PC-SIDE), Version 1.02.* ISU, Ames.

Jago, R., J. S. Harrell, R. G. McMurray, S. Edelstein, L. El Ghormli, and S. Bassin. 2006. Prevalence of abnormal lipid and blood pressure values among an ethnically diverse population of eighth-grade adolescents and screening implications. *Pediatrics* 117(6):2065–2073.

Koebnick, C., N. Smith, K. J. Coleman, D. Getahun, K. Reynolds, V. P. Quinn, A. H. Porter, J. K. Der-Sarkissian, and S. J. Jacobsen. 2010. Prevalence of extreme obesity in a multiethnic cohort of children and adolescents. *Journal of Pediatrics* 157(1):26–31.c2.

Kuczmarski, R. J., C. L. Ogden, L. M. Grummer-Strawn, K. M. Flegal, S. S. Guo, R. Wei, Z. Mei, L. R. Curtin, A. F. Roche, and C. L. Johnson. 2000. CDC growth charts: United States. *Advance Data from Vital and Health Statistics* (314):1–28, http://www.cdc.gov/nchs/data/ad/ad314.pdf (accessed July 28, 2009).

Messiah, S. E., K. L. Arheart, B. Luke, S. E. Lipshultz, and T. L. Miller. 2008. Relationship between body mass index and metabolic syndrome risk factors among U.S. 8- to 14-year-olds, 1999 to 2002. *Journal of Pediatrics* 153(2):215–221.

NCHS (National Center for Health Statistics). 2007. *Prevalence of Overweight, Infants and Children Less Than 2 Years of Age: United States, 2003–2004.* http://www.cdc.gov/nchs/data/hestat/overweight/overweight_child_under02.htm (accessed March 11, 2010).

Ogden, C. L., M. D. Carroll, L. R. Curtin, M. A. McDowell, C. J. Tabak, and K. M. Flegal. 2006. Prevalence of overweight and obesity in the United States, 1999–2004. *Journal of the American Medical Association* 295(13):1549–1555.

Ogden, C. L., M. D. Carroll, and K. M. Flegal. 2008. High body mass index for age among U.S. children and adolescents, 2003–2006. *Journal of the American Medical Association* 299(20):2401–2405.

Ogden, C. L., M. D. Carroll, L. R. Curtin, M. M. Lamb, and K. M. Flegal. 2010. Prevalence of high body mass index in US children and adolescents, 2007–2008. *Journal of the American Medical Association* 303(3):242–249.

Skinner, J. D., P. Ziegler, and M. Ponza. 2004. Transitions in infants' and toddlers' beverage patterns. *Journal of the American Dietetic Association* 104(Suppl. 1):S45–S50.

USDA/ARS (U.S. Department of Agriculture/Agricultural Research Service). 2000. *1994–1996 Continuing Survey of Food Intakes by Individuals (CSFII 1994–1996) and 1998 Supplemental Children's Survey (CSFII 1998).* Beltsville, MD: ARS.

USDA/ARS. 2009. *What We Eat in America, NHANES 2005–2006: Usual Nutrient Intakes from Food and Water Compared to 1997 Dietary Reference Intakes for Vitamin D, Calcium, Phosphorus, and Magnesium.* Washington, DC: USDA/ARS.

USDA/FCS (U.S. Department of Agriculture/Food and Consumer Service). 1997. *WIC Infant Feeding Practices Study. Final Report.* Alexandria, VA: USDA/FCS. http://www.fns.usda.gov/oane/menu/published/wic/files/wicifps.pdf (accessed July 12, 2010).

USDA/FNS (U.S. Department of Agriculture/Food and Nutrition Service). 2008. *Diet Quality of American School-Age Children by School Lunch Participation Status: Data from the National Health and Nutrition Examination Survey, 1999–2004.* Alexandria, VA: USDA/FNS. http://www.fns.usda.gov/OANE/menu/published/CNP/FILES/NHANES-NSLP.pdf (accessed August 20, 2008).

USDA/HHS (U.S. Department of Agriculture/U.S. Department of Health and Human Services). 2010. *Report of the Dietary Guidelines Advisory Committee on the Dietary Guidelines for Americans, 2010.* http://www.cnpp.usda.gov/DGAs2010-DGACReport.htm (accessed June 29, 2010).

Vatanparast, H., D. A. Bailey, A. D. G. Baxter-Jones, and S. J. Whiting. 2010. Calcium requirements for bone growth in Canadian boys and girls during adolescence. *British Journal of Nutrition* 103 (4):575–580.

Weaver, C. M., and R. P. Heaney. 2006. Calcium. In *Modern Nutrition in Health and Disease*, edited by M. E. Shils, M. Shike, A. C. Ross, B. Caballero and R. J. Cousins. Philadelphia, PA: Lippincott, Williams, and Wilkins.

Weiss, R., and S. Caprio. 2005. The metabolic consequences of childhood obesity. *Best Practice and Research: Clinical Endocrinology and Metabolism* 19(3):405–419.

Ziegler, P., R. Briefel, N. Clusen, and B. Devaney. 2006. Feeding Infants and Toddlers Study (FITS): Development of the FITS survey in comparison to other dietary survey methods. *Journal of the American Dietetic Association* 106(1 Suppl):S12–S27.

5

Nutritional Considerations for Adults

To provide a basis for recommending revisions to the meal requirements of the Child and Adult Care Food Program (CACFP), this chapter presents the committee's findings regarding food and nutrient intakes by adults. First it relates the findings regarding food intake for two adult age groups to the current *Dietary Guidelines for Americans* (DGA) (HHS/USDA, 2005) and MyPyramid food guide (USDA, 2010). Then it presents nutrient intakes in relation to selected types of Dietary Reference Intakes (DRIs). The chapter includes special nutritional considerations relating to meeting the needs for vitamins B_{12} and D, chronic disease, texture modifications, and recognizing the influence of ethnic and religious tradition on food choices. The chapter ends with the identification of key foods and nutrients that should be either encouraged or limited. To examine intakes, the committee used the data sets, other source materials, and methods that are described in Chapter 3.

FOOD INTAKES

Most adult participants in CACFP are over the age of 60 years, but younger adults (19–59 years of age) may participate in CACFP if they have disabilities that require them to be in a supervised setting (see Chapter 2). Thus, the committee considered these two age groups separately when comparing food group intake to the amounts specified by MyPyramid for a 2,000-calorie intake level. Although it is recognized that calorie requirements vary greatly among adult men and women, the committee arrived at a 2,000-calorie level for meal planning purposes. It is the closest

MyPyramid level to the mean of the total energy expenditure for the four age groups in the National Health and Nutrition Examination Survey (NHANES) 2003–2004: men and women, ages 19–59 years and 60 years or older, when body mass index was imputed at 22.5 for the younger and at 25 for the older group of adults (see Chapter 3). Because of the variation in available facilities in adult day care programs, it was not considered practical to set different calorie levels for subgroups at the meal planning stage. It should be noted, however, that portion sizes may be adjusted within facilities, as appropriate.

The data in Table 5-1 show the areas that mean adult intakes of all the food groups and subgroups were below the MyPyramid amounts, with the exception of total grains for the 19–59-year age group. For both age groups, mean fruit intake was only about half of the amount that would be consistent with the MyPyramid pattern. Furthermore, within the vegetables group, the consumption of dark green vegetables, orange vegetables, and dried beans and peas was lower than the MyPyramid amount specified for each of these individual subgroups. Neither age group approached the recommended amount of whole grains.

Note that the 2005 DGA (HHS/USDA, 2005) encourages the intake of increased amounts of a variety of vegetables and fruits and recommends that at least half of the grain be whole grain. In addition to providing nutrients, fruits and vegetables provide numerous beneficial phytochemicals, which may be protective of a wide variety of age-related conditions (Carlsen et al., 2010). The 2010 Dietary Guidelines Advisory Committee (USDA/HHS, 2010) placed strong emphasis on a diet that is primarily plant-based—rich in vegetables, fruits, whole grains, nuts, and seeds.

Meeting the nutrient needs of older and disabled adults with lower calorie requirements poses great challenges in the context of the typical American diet. As seen in the analyses above, calories from solid fats and added sugars for the general adult population far exceed caloric requirements. Placing limits on energy-dense foods such as fatty meats, full-fat dairy products, sugar-sweetened drinks, and pastries and other desserts can reduce the intake of solid fat, sugars, and calories. This change makes room for more vegetables, fruits, whole grains, and low-fat or nonfat fluid milk and milk products without providing excess calories.

ENERGY AND NUTRIENT INTAKES

Energy

The committee considered estimated energy intakes by adults as discussed in Chapter 3.

TABLE 5-1 Comparison Between the 2,000-Calorie MyPyramid Food Group Pattern and Mean Daily Amounts of MyPyramid Food Groups Consumed by Adults ≥ 19 Years of Age

Food Group or Component[b]	Age Group		
	≥ 19 Years	19–59 Years[a]	≥ 60 Years[a]
	2,000 kcal Pattern	Mean Intake	Mean Intake
Total fruit (cup eq)	2	0.96	1.13
Total vegetables (cup eq)	2.5	1.77	1.65
Dark green	0.43[c]	0.10	0.11
Orange	0.29[c]	0.07	0.09
Dry beans/peas	0.43[c]	0.13	0.13
Starchy	0.43[c]	0.50	0.47
Other	0.93[c]	0.97	0.85
Total grains (oz eq)	6	7.11	5.83
Whole grains (oz eq)	3	0.61	0.86
Total meat and beans (oz eq)[d]	5.5	5.19	4.08
Total milk group (8 fl oz eq)[e]	3	1.67	1.33
Vegetable oils (g)[f]	27	21	17
SoFAS (kcal)	267	804[g]	570[g]

NOTES: The MyPyramid food intake pattern used is from the *Dietary Guidelines for Americans* (HHS/USDA, 2005). Eq = equivalent; fl = fluid; g = gram; kcal = calories; oz = ounce; SoFAS = solid fats and added sugars.

[a]Average of male and female intake data.

[b]See Appendix Table H-1 for a list of foods in the MyPyramid food groups and subgroups.

[c]Daily amounts based on the MyPyramid recommendations expressed as cup equivalents per week.

[d]The MyPyramid meat and beans group includes meat, poultry, fish, eggs, dry beans and peas, and nuts and seeds (http://www.mypyramid.gov/pyramid/meat.html).

[e]The MyPyramid milk group includes fluid milk; hard, soft, and processed cheese; yogurt; and milk-based desserts (http://www.mypyramid.gov/pyramid/milk.html). The intake data represent mean intake of fluid milk, cheese, and yogurt. *Dietary Guidelines* advises "3 cups per day of fat-free or low-fat milk or equivalent milk products" for adults (see HHS/USDA, 2005, p. viii).

[f]5 g = 1 teaspoon.

[g]Estimated on the basis of the number of grams of discretionary solid fat and the number of teaspoons (tsp) of added sugars, as follows: (fat g × 9 calories/g) + (tsp × 4.2 g/tsp × 4 calories/g).

SOURCES: Mean intake data from NHANES 2003–2004; MyPyramid patterns from Britten et al., 2006.

Nutrients with an Estimated Average Requirement

The committee examined nutrient intakes by adults in relation to selected DRIs to identify nutrients for which intake is likely to be inadequate or excessive. To do this, the committee conducted analyses of dietary intake data from the NHANES 2003–2004 survey (CDC, 2010). Table 5-2 shows the estimated prevalence of inadequate usual intakes for nutrients that have an Estimated Average Requirement (EAR), by gender and age group.

Consistent with other reports, this analysis of NHANES (2003–2004) data (see Table 5-2) shows that older adults (> 60 years of age) are at greater risk than younger adults for inadequate intakes for several nutrients. Very few individuals of any age achieve adequate vitamin E intakes. For both age groups, the prevalence of inadequate intakes of vitamins A and C and magnesium exceeds 40 percent; that of zinc ranges from 8 to 26 percent; and all but younger men show a prevalence of inadequate intakes of vitamin B_6, folate, and thiamin that range from 6 to 39 percent. Women in both age groups appear to be more likely than men to have a high prevalence of inadequate intakes of protein, thiamin, vitamin B_6, folate, and vitamin B_{12}. Iron is a concern only for adult women of child-bearing age. Low protein intake may be of particular concern for older adults because, compared with younger adults, they have lower efficiency of protein utili-

TABLE 5-2 Estimated Prevalence of Inadequacy of Protein and Selected Vitamins and Minerals Among Adults Based on Usual Nutrient Intakes from NHANES 2003–2004[a]

| | Estimated Prevalence of Inadequate Usual Intakes (%) by Age Group (years) and Gender | | | |
| | 19–59 Years | | ≥ 60 Years | |
	Males	Females	Males	Females
Protein	3.4	**14**	**12**	**20**
Vitamin A	**54**	**54**	**54**	**43**
Vitamin C	**44**	**40**	**49**	**40**
Vitamin E	**89**	**97**	**92**	**98**
Thiamin	1.6	**9**	**6**	**12**
Riboflavin	0.8	3.3	2.8	3.7
Niacin	0.2	2.1	1.8	4.6
Vitamin B_6	4.2	**21**	**19**	**39**
Folate	3.2	**17**	**11**	**24**
Vitamin B_{12}	0.9	**7**	2.4	**9**
Phosphorus	0.2	2.4	1.2	4.8
Magnesium	**57**	**65**	**78**	**73**
Iron	0.1	**12**	1.0	1.5
Zinc	**8**	**12**	**26**	**21**

NOTE: Bold font indicates values with a prevalence of inadequacy greater than 5 percent.

[a]All nutrients in this table have an Estimated Average Requirement (EAR).

SOURCES: Intake data from NHANES 2003–2004. The EARs used in the analysis were from the Dietary Reference Intake reports (IOM, 1997, 1998, 2000, 2001, 2002/2005).

zation, and they tend to lose lean body mass over time (Gaffney-Stomberg et al., 2009).

Selected Nutrients with an Adequate Intake

Intakes of selected nutrients that have an Adequate Intake (AI) rather than an EAR are shown in Table 5-3, by age group and gender, along with the respective AI. The mean and median NHANES (2003–2004) intakes for calcium, potassium, and fiber are lower than the AI for most of these adult age-gender groups, suggesting that the majority of individuals do not meet this target recommendation. Women have lower intakes than do men, with mean and median potassium intakes less than half the α-linoleic and α-linolenic acid intakes are close to the AI on average.

TABLE 5-3 Comparison Between Median Nutrient Intakes from NHANES (2003–2004) and the Adequate Intake (AI), by Age Group (in years) and Gender

	19–59 Years		≥ 60 Years	
	Males	Females	Males	Females
Calcium (mg/d)				
AI	1,044	1,044	1,200	1,200
Mean intake	1,068	**790**	**846**	**702**
Median intake	1,003	758	798	654
Potassium (mg/d)				
AI	4,700	4,700	4,700	4,700
Mean intake	**3,182**	**2,342**	**2,866**	**2,327**
Median intake	3,112	2,292	2,787	2,290
Fiber (g/d)				
AI	36.2	24.1	30.0	21.0
Mean intake	**17.3**	**13.4**	**16.4**	**13.8**
Median intake	16.3	12.7	15.7	13.4
Linoleic acid (g/d)				
AI	16.3	11.8	14.0	11.0
Mean intake	18.8	14.2	15.1	12.3
Median intake	17.9	13.4	14.2	11.5
α-linolenic acid (g/d)				
AI	1.6	1.1	1.6	1.1
Mean intake	1.9	1.4	**1.5**	**1.3**
Median intake	1.8	1.3	1.4	1.2

NOTES: AI = Adequate Intake; g/d = grams per day; mg/d = milligrams per day. Bold font indicates mean intake values lower than the AI.
SOURCES: Intake data from NHANES 2003–2004. The AIs used in the analysis were from the DRI reports (IOM, 1997, 2002/2005, 2005). AIs shown for the 19–59-year-old age group are weighted averages of two DRI age groups.

Data from *What We Eat in America*, NHANES 2007–2008 (USDA/ARS, 2010, Table 1), indicate that mean vitamin D intake by adult males ages 20 years or older is at the AI of 5.0 μg, but it is below the AI for those ages 60 years or older. For all adult females, mean vitamin D intake is well below the AI.

Excessive Intake Levels

The Tolerable Upper Intake Level for sodium is 2.3 g per day for adults. Reported mean sodium intake is substantially higher for adult males (4.4 g per day) than for adult females (3.1 g per day) (IOM, 2010). The 2010 Dietary Guidelines Advisory Committee (USDA/HHS, 2010) recommended gradual movement toward an even lower maximum sodium intake—1.5 g per day.

On average, data from NHANES show that both male and female adults have intakes of saturated fat that exceed 10 percent of total calories (USDA/ARS, 2010, Table 5)—the maximum proportion of saturated fat calories recommended in the 2005 DGA (HHS/USDA, 2005). The 2010 Dietary Guidelines Advisory Committee (USDA/HHS, 2010) recommended intake of less than 10 percent of total calories from saturated fat as an interim step toward reaching a goal of less than 7 percent of total calories from saturated fat.

NHANES data also show that cholesterol intake differs substantially by gender (higher for males than for females) and age (starting to decrease at about age 50). On average, males ages 20–69 years have a mean cholesterol intake that exceeds 300 mg per day, whereas mean intakes are below 300 mg per day for adult women and for men ages 70 years and older (USDA/ARS, 2010, Table 1).

SPECIAL NUTRITIONAL CONSIDERATIONS

The nutrient comparisons in Tables 5-2 and 5-3 are based on the noninstitutionalized U.S. adult population. However, the committee recognizes that the nutritional concerns of adults who are receiving day care in group homes or centers are not necessarily typical of free-living adults of the same age who can care for themselves. Inadequate intakes are likely more severe in this population, while the demands of chronic conditions and medications may increase the need for some nutrients. Disability and functional dependence, which are characteristic of adults in day care, often are related to disease. Disability in older men is usually related to heart disease and stroke; disability in older women is usually associated with osteoporosis and related fractures, arthritis, and circulatory diseases (Fried and Guralnik, 1997; La Croix et al., 1997). Some individuals entering adult day care may have compromised nutritional status because they have had limited access to food. Tooth loss, infection, lesions, and other oral problems are prevalent in older adults and, if present, will contribute to altered dietary intake. Younger adults who participate in CACFP have various disabilities that may affect their nutritional status and functionality.

Vitamins B_{12} and D

Vitamin B_{12}

Vitamin B_{12} merits special attention. Even though Table 5-2 shows that the prevalence of vitamin B_{12} inadequacy is less than 3 percent for males and 7 to 9 percent for females, vitamin B_{12} deficiency may be more prevalent than this. The discrepancy between the apparent prevalence of inadequacy and actual deficiency relates to the absorption of protein-bound vitamin B_{12} by individuals over the age of 50 years. Ten to 30 percent of this older population may suffer from some degree of atrophic gastritis, leading to a decrease in stomach acid (IOM, 1998). Lack of gastric acid, in turn, leads to decreased absorption of the vitamin B_{12} provided by animal foods. For this reason, the Institute of Medicine recommends that older adults obtain their Recommended Dietary Allowance (RDA) of vitamin B_{12} mainly in the crystalline form, as from fortified foods (e.g., fortified breakfast cereals) or supplements (IOM, 1998). Data from *What We Eat in America* (USDA/ARS, 2010, Table 1) indicate that the mean daily intake of added (crystalline) vitamin B_{12} in fortified foods by adults ages 20 years and older was about 1 µg per day—far less than the RDA of 2.4 µg.

Vitamin D and Calcium

Elderly adults tend to have poor dairy and vitamin D intake, decreased sun exposure as well as reduced dermal synthesis of $1,25\text{-}OH_2\text{-}D$, and secondary hyperparathyroidism, all of which contribute to increased risk for poor bone health and fracture risk in this population. Concentrations of provitamin D_3 in the epidermis are inversely related to age (MacLaughlin and Holick, 1985), which results in decreased production of vitamin D from sunlight exposure. Estimates of vitamin D synthesis in elderly adults suggest about a 70 percent decrease in the elderly compared to young adults (Holick et al., 1989). In women, bone loss occurs as a result of low estrogen levels that accompany menopause and the combined effects of other age-related changes on vitamin D and calcium metabolism. Estrogen has a regulatory role in synthesis of $1,25\text{-}OH_2\text{-}D$ (Caniggia et al., 1987), and the reduction of estrogen as a result of menopause is correlated with a progressive increase in parathyroid hormone, which in turn increases bone turnover and risk for osteoporosis (Khosla et al., 1997). Adequate vitamin D intake in this population is important to reduce secondary hyperparathyroidism and its attendant effects on bone turnover (Gennari, 2001).

Low Level of Physical Activity

Because of their disability or for other reasons, adults attending day care may be more sedentary than the general population. An analysis of data from the Behavioral Risk Factor Surveillance System found that noninstitutionalized adults with disability do not meet basic recommendations for physical activity according to recommendations from the Centers for Disease Control and Prevention and the American College of Sports Medicine (Boslaugh and Andresen, 2006). Messent et al. (1999) identified several barriers to activity encountered by individuals with learning disabilities. These included "unclear policy guidelines in residential and day service provision together with resourcing, transport and staffing constraints; participant income and expenditure; and limited options for physically active community leisure" (p. 409). An increase in physical activity may improve appetite and allow the consumption of additional food without leading to weight gain.

Impact of Chronic Disease

Any chronic disease may affect an individual's nutrient needs or otherwise have an impact on nutritional status. Dietary modifications, which are described briefly below, may be needed to support health, and medications may affect dietary intake or lead to drug-nutrient interactions. Conditions that may require dietary modifications include obesity, frailty, hypertension, type 2 diabetes, and heart disease. Adequate nutrition and good dietary quality for individuals with these conditions may reduce morbidity and mortality.

Obesity is associated with disability among older adults (Houston et al., 2009). Weight gain may contribute to disability by making it more difficult to maintain activity levels and mobility (Rolland et al., 2009; Zamboni et al., 2008). Disability has been associated with a myriad of syndromes including malnutrition, inflammatory disease (especially in persons with multiple chronic conditions), and functional dependency (Becker, 1994; Topinková, 2008). For these reasons, among others, it is especially important for the meals and snacks provided to adults in day care to support healthy weight while providing adequate levels of nutrients.

Modified Diets

In many cases, adults with chronic disease may be prescribed a special diet. Some larger adult day care centers have access to a professional kitchen and a dietitian and can accommodate these needs as directed by each person's health care provider. Smaller centers and group homes may need more assistance in meeting these needs. The most commonly prescribed modifications include lowering sodium, dietary fat, and total calories. For most of the chronic conditions that may result in a need for day care, these modifications are consistent with the *Dietary Guidelines* and can be accommodated with a general menu, thereby limiting the need for highly specialized individual meals. It should be noted that the American Dietetic Association has long recommended liberalized diets for older adults (ADA, 2005). Consideration of unique special dietary needs is beyond the scope of the committee's charge. Therefore, the committee focused on the majority of older adults and adults with disabilities who may or may not have common chronic conditions, all of whom are likely to benefit from a diet that follows the *Dietary Guidelines*.

Functional Limitations

Adults of any age who have functional limitations often need assistance with eating and drinking. Measures described below may be necessary to ensure that adequate food and fluid can be consumed regardless of whether the person can eat independently or is fed by a care provider, relative, or friend.

Providing Adequate Fluid

Meeting fluid requirements may be challenging for the functionally disabled and for older adults. Regardless of age, some disabled adults are unable to drink fluids without assistance, and some may want to restrict fluid intake to reduce the need to urinate. As individuals age, thirst sensitivity decreases; many older adults do not have the trigger initiated by a normal thirst mechanism to consume fluids. The frequent offering of small amounts of beverages helps such individuals meet their need for fluids.

Modifying Textures

Textures may be modified to accommodate oral health problems, including but not limited to loose teeth, oral lesions, and gum and periodontal disease. Modifications in texture also may be necessary to accommodate swallowing difficulties that occur because of chronic disease (e.g., Parkinson's disease) or catastrophic illness (e.g., stroke, cancer). Examples of texture modifications include the dicing, mincing, pureeing, and liquefying of foods and the thickening of liquids.

Recognizing Ethnic and Religious Traditions

Many older people have food consumption habits that are from familial and ethnic traditions, and these food habits may not mirror present-day dietary recommendations. Recognizing the importance of maintaining ethnic, religious, and other food patterns is very important, however. Redeveloping recipes for ethnic foods that may be more healthful has been a successful strategy.

FOODS AND NUTRIENTS TO BE ENCOURAGED OR LIMITED

The analyses of food and nutrient intakes by adults make it clear that special effort will be needed to both provide and encourage intake of more fruit, vegetables, low-fat dairy products, and whole grains while limiting exposure to and the consumption of foods high in sugar, solid fats, and sodium and of refined grains. Greater intake of fruit and vegetables will improve intake of vitamin C, carotenoids (dark green and orange vegetables), folate (dark green vegetables, oranges, and legumes), vitamin B_6 (legumes and bananas), magnesium (legumes), potassium, and dietary fiber (most nonstarchy fruits and vegetables). Higher intakes of low-fat milk or yogurt will improve intakes of magnesium, calcium, potassium, vitamin B_{12}, and, if fortified, vitamin D. Inclusion of fortified breakfast cereals will provide some crystalline vitamin B_{12}. The inclusion of more whole grains will improve intakes of vitamin B_6, magnesium, and dietary fiber.

REFERENCES

ADA (American Dietetic Association). 2005. Position of the American Dietetic Association: Liberalization of the diet prescription improves quality of life for older adults in long-term care. *Journal of the American Dietetic Association* 105(12):1955–1965.

Becker, G. 1994. The oldest old: Autonomy in the face of frailty. *Journal of Aging Studies* 8(1):59–76.

Boslaugh, S. E., and E. M. Andresen. 2006. Correlates of physical activity for adults with disability. *Preventing Chronic Disease* 3(3):A78.

Britten, P., K. Marcoe, S. Yamini, and C. Davis. 2006. Development of food intake patterns for the MyPyramid Food Guidance System. *Journal of Nutrition Education and Behavior* 38(6 Suppl):S78–S92.

Caniggia, A., F. Lore, G. di Cairano, and R. Nuti. 1987. Main endocrine modulators of vitamin D hydroxylases in human pathophysiology. *Journal of Steroid Biochemistry* 27(4–6):815–824.

Carlsen, M. H., B. L. Halvorsen, K. Holte, S. K. Bøhn, S. Dragland, L. Sampson, C. Willey, H. Senoo, Y. Umezono, C. Sanada, I. Barikmo, N. Berhe, W. C. Willett, K. M. Phillips, D. R. Jacobs, and R. Blomhoff. 2010. The total antioxidant content of more than 3100 foods, beverages, spices, herbs and supplements used worldwide. *Nutrition Journal* 9(1):Article No. 3.

CDC (Centers for Disease Control and Prevention). 2010. *NHANES 2003–2004.* http://www. cdc.gov/nchs/nhanes/nhanes2003-2004/nhanes03_04.htm (accessed August 18, 2010)

Fried, L. P., and J. M. Guralnik. 1997. Disability in older adults: Evidence regarding significance, etiology, and risk. *Journal of the American Geriatrics Society* 45(1):92–100.

Gaffney-Stomberg, E., K. L. Insogna, N. R. Rodriguez, and J. E. Kerstetter. 2009. Increasing dietary protein requirements in elderly people for optimal muscle and bone health. *Journal of the American Geriatrics Society* 57(6):1073–1079.

Gennari, C. 2001. Calcium and vitamin D nutrition and bone disease of the elderly. *Public Health Nutrition* 4(2 B):547–559.

HHS/USDA (U.S. Department of Health and Human Services/U.S. Department of Agriculture). 2005. *Dietary Guidelines for Americans,* 6th ed. Washington, DC: U.S. Government Printing Office. http://www.health.gov/DietaryGuidelines/dga2005/document/ (accessed July 23, 2008).

Holick, M. F., L. Y. Matsuoka, and J. Wortsman. 1989. Age, vitamin D, and solar ultraviolet. *Lancet* 334(8671):1104–1105.

Houston, D. K., B. J. Nicklas, and C. A. Zizza. 2009. Weighty concerns: The growing prevalence of obesity among older adults. *Journal of the American Dietetic Association* 109(11):1886–1895.

IOM (Institute of Medicine). 1997. *Dietary Reference Intakes for Calcium, Phosphorus, Magnesium, Vitamin D, and Fluoride.* Washington, DC: National Academy Press.

IOM. 1998. *Dietary Reference Intakes for Thiamin, Riboflavin, Niacin, Vitamin B₆, Folate, Vitamin B₁₂, Pantothenic Acid, Biotin, and Choline.* Washington, DC: National Academy Press.

IOM. 2000. *Dietary Reference Intakes for Vitamin C, Vitamin E, Selenium, and Carotenoids.* Washington, DC: National Academy Press.

IOM. 2001. *Dietary Reference Intakes for Vitamin A, Vitamin K, Arsenic, Boron, Chromium, Copper, Iodine, Iron, Manganese, Molybdenum, Nickel, Silicon, Vanadium, and Zinc.* Washington, DC: National Academy Press.

IOM. 2002/2005. *Dietary Reference Intakes for Energy, Carbohydrate, Fiber, Fat, Fatty Acids, Cholesterol, Protein, and Amino Acids.* Washington, DC: The National Academies Press.

IOM. 2005. *Dietary Reference Intakes for Water, Potassium, Sodium, Chloride, and Sulfate.* Washington, DC: The National Academies Press.

IOM. 2010. *Strategies to Reduce Sodium Intake in the United States.* Washington, DC: The National Academies Press.

Khosla, S., E. J. Atkinson, L. J. Melton III, and B. L. Riggs. 1997. Effects of age and estrogen status on serum parathyroid hormone levels and biochemical markers of bone turnover in women: A population-based study. *Journal of Clinical Endocrinology and Metabolism* 82(5):1522–1527.

La Croix, A. Z., K. M. Newton, S. G. Leveille, and J. Wallace. 1997. Healthy aging: A women's issue. *Western Journal of Medicine* 167(4):220–232.

MacLaughlin, J., and M. F. Holick. 1985. Aging decreases the capacity of human skin to produce vitamin D₃. *Journal of Clinical Investigation* 76(4):1536–1538.

Messent, P. R., C. B. Cooke, and J. Long. 1999. Primary and secondary barriers to physically active healthy lifestyles for adults with learning disabilities. *Disability and Rehabilitation* 21(9):409–419.

Rolland, Y., V. Lauwers-Cances, C. Cristini, G. A. Van Kan, I. Janssen, J. E. Morley, and B. Vellas. 2009. Difficulties with physical function associated with obesity, sarcopenia, and sarcopenic-obesity in community-dwelling elderly women: The EPIDOS (EPIDemiologie de l'OSteoporose) Study. *American Journal of Clinical Nutrition* 89(6):1895–1900.

Topinková, E. 2008. Aging, disability and frailty. *Annals of Nutrition and Metabolism* 52(Suppl 1):6–11.

USDA (U.S. Department of Agriculture). 2010. *MyPyramid.* http://www.mypyramid.gov/ (accessed June 29, 2010).

USDA/ARS (U.S. Department of Agriculture/Agricultural Research Service). 2010. *What We Eat in America, NHANES 2007–2008.* http://www.ars.usda.gov/Services/docs. htm?docid=18349 (accessed October 5, 2010).

USDA/HHS (U.S. Department of Agriculture/U.S. Department of Health and Human Services). 2010. *Report of the Dietary Guidelines Advisory Committee on the Dietary Guidelines for Americans, 2010.* http://www.cnpp.usda.gov/DGAs2010-DGACReport.htm (accessed June 29, 2010).

Zamboni, M., G. Mazzali, F. Fantin, A. Rossi, and V. Di Francesco. 2008. Sarcopenic obesity: A new category of obesity in the elderly. *Nutrition, Metabolism and Cardiovascular Diseases* 18(5):388–395.

6

Process for Developing Recommendations for Meal Requirements

This chapter describes the approach the committee used in developing recommendations for revisions to Meal Requirements for the Child and Adult Care Food Program (CACFP). The bulk of this chapter describes the processes used in developing recommendations for Meal Requirements for children over the age of 1 year, adolescents, and adults. The process that was used in developing recommendations for infants is described at the end of the chapter. A comparison of the consistency of the recommended Meal Requirements with the committee's criteria is provided in Chapter 10.

CRITERIA

To guide its work the committee developed a set of criteria, shown in Box 6-1. These criteria provided an overarching framework that the committee used in developing, evaluating, and finalizing its recommendations.

OVERALL APPROACH TO DEVELOPING RECOMMENDATIONS

The committee's approach to developing recommendations for CACFP Meal Requirements for children ages 1–18 years and adults ages 19 years and older was based on the approach used by the Committee on Nutrition Standards for the National School Lunch and Breakfast Programs (hereafter called the School Meals committee) (IOM, 2010). The process included several steps:

BOX 6-1
CACFP Criteria

Criterion 1. The Meal Requirements will be consistent with current dietary guidance and nutrition recommendations to promote health with the ultimate goal of improving participants' diets by reducing the prevalence of inadequate and excessive intakes of food, nutrients, and calories.
  a. For infants and children younger than 2 years of age, the Meal Requirements will contribute to an overall diet that is consistent with established dietary recommendations for this age group and encourage and support breastfeeding for infants.
  b. For participating adults and children ages 2 years and older, the Meal Requirements will be consistent with the *Dietary Guidelines for Americans* and the Dietary Reference Intakes.

Criterion 2. The Meal Requirements will provide the basis for menus that are practical to plan, purchase, prepare, and serve in different settings.

Criterion 3. The Meal Requirements will provide the basis for menus that incorporate healthful foods and beverages and are appealing to diverse age ranges and cultural backgrounds.

Criterion 4. The Meal Requirements will facilitate the planning of menus that are compatible with the capabilities and resources for the variety of program providers.

Criterion 5. The Meal Requirements will allow the planning of menus that are sensitive to considerations of cost.

---

1. Set age groups and total daily mean calorie requirements for each group. The methods used to initially set these parameters are described in the section "The Determination of Age Groups, Body Weights and Heights, and Estimated Calorie Requirements" in Chapter 3. The final age groups used for developing the Meal Requirements reflect the committee's decision to combine groups with similar nutrient and calorie requirements. The final age groups are shown in Table 6-1.
2. Assess dietary intakes and consider relevant laboratory data and health effects of inadequate or excessive intakes to identify the food and nutrient intakes of concern for specified age groups. Dietary intakes included food groups, food subgroups, calories, and nutrients. Chapter 3 presents the methods used to examine intakes. These methods are consistent with those recommended by the

Institute of Medicine (2000). Chapter 4 presents the findings for infants and children, and Chapter 5 presents the findings for adults.

3. Develop calorie and nutrient targets for each meal and snack. In developing these targets, the committee used methods recommended in the report *Dietary Reference Intakes: Applications in Dietary Planning* (IOM, 2003) when applicable. The targets are described later in this chapter.

4. Develop meal patterns and food specifications for planning meals and snacks that are aligned with the nutrient targets and the *Dietary Guidelines*. Apply the criteria (Box 6-1) in an iterative fashion to evaluate and finalize the recommended Meal Requirements. The recommendations are presented in Chapter 7.

Figure 6-1 illustrates the process used by the committee in developing its recommendations for revisions to existing Meal Requirements for CACFP. The boxes and pathway in the center of the figure depict the major components of the committee's approach. The boxes on the right and the left show the elements that were considered or evaluated as the committee applied its criteria to evolving recommendations.

The double arrows and dashed lines indicate the iterative steps in the process. For example, initial proposals for the Meal Requirements were evaluated to determine how well they aligned with current dietary guidance and were modified as necessary to enhance this consistency. Similar evaluations were undertaken to assess the practicality of proposed Meal Requirements as well as their suitability for use in planning menus that are consistent with the capabilities and resources of program providers.

After preliminary Meal Requirements were specified, two approaches were used to evaluate them. The first involved the development of meal composites that were revised to reflect the preliminary Meal Requirements (see "Development of Composite Food Items and Groups for Recommended Meal Requirements" in Appendix I). The second involved the writing of sample menus based on the Meal Requirements. Both the revised

TABLE 6-1 Age Groups Used to Develop CACFP Meal Requirements

Population Group	Age Range
Infants	0–5 months
	6–11 months
Children	1 year
	2–4 years
	5–13 years
Adolescents	14–18 years
Adults	$\geq$ 19 years

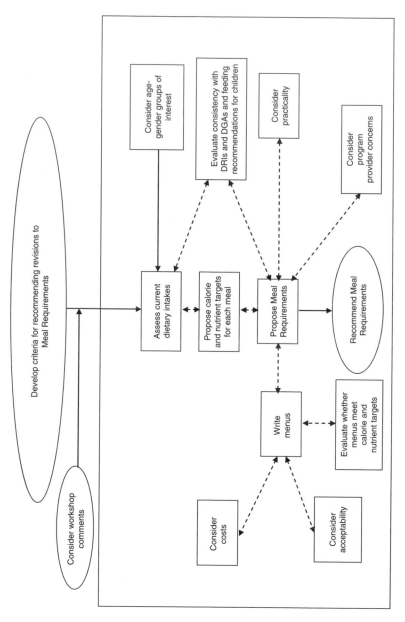

FIGURE 6-1 Process for revising current Nutrition Standards and Meal Requirements for the Child and Adult Care Food Program. Dashed lines indicate the iterative nature of the process.
NOTES: DGA = Dietary Guidelines for Americans; DRI = Dietary Reference Intake.

meal composites and the menus were evaluated for cost and correspondence with the nutrient targets. The menus were also evaluated for acceptability and practicality. This resulted in some changes in the preliminary Meal Requirements. The end product of this iterative process was a set of recommendations for CACFP Meal Requirements.

ESTABLISHING CALORIE AND NUTRIENT TARGETS

The committee developed targets for calories and 24 nutrients and other dietary components for each of the seven specified age groups. These targets served as a guide for developing the new Meal Requirements and helped ensure that they would align well with the Dietary Reference Intakes (DRIs) (IOM, 1997, 1998, 2000, 2001, 2002/2005, 2005) and the 2005 *Dietary Guidelines* (HHS/USDA, 2005). In setting the targets, the committee used the approach developed and implemented by the School Meals committee (IOM, 2010). As described below, different approaches were used to develop targets for (1) calories, (2) nutrients with Estimated Average Requirements (EARs), (3) nutrients with Adequate Intakes (AIs), and (4) macronutrients. The targets vary by age group and eating occasion.

Calorie Targets

Estimated Energy Requirements

Before nutrient targets could be set for CACFP meals and snacks, it was essential to determine appropriate calorie targets. To do this, the committee first estimated the average daily energy requirements of several age groups of children and adults served by CACFP (see Chapter 3, Table 3-3). The committee used rounded overall means in setting calorie targets for specific meals and snacks and in other calculations related to the Meal Requirements. Of necessity, these calorie levels will be too high for some subgroups (mainly adolescent and older adult females) and too low for others. In using the overall mean, the committee sought to achieve a satisfactory balance between these two extremes, recognizing that gender-specific calorie targets are impractical for use in a group feeding program. As explained in the section "Food Intakes" in Chapter 5, adults ages 19 years and older were considered a single group with a daily calorie target of 2,000 calories per day. Likewise, the 5–10- and 11–13-year age groups were combined, and a mean calorie level of 1,900 calories per day was used in the analyses.

Distribution of Calories Across Eating Occasions

As a first step in setting target calorie levels for CACFP meals and snacks, the committee analyzed data from the National Health and Nutrition Examination Survey (NHANES) 2003–2004 to determine, for each of six age groups, the average proportion of total daily calories consumed at breakfast, lunch, and dinner by individuals who reported these eating occasions. Results of this analysis are summarized in Table 6-2. After summing the percentage of calories consumed at the three meals, the remaining percentage was calculated and assumed to be available for consumption as snacks. On average, children and adults consume approximately 22 percent of their total daily calorie intake at breakfast, 31 percent at lunch, 35 percent at dinner, and the remainder in snacks. Compared with the other age groups, however, the youngest children (ages 1–4 years) consume a lower percentage of their calories at meals and a higher percentage at snacks. This reflects the fact that children in this age range tend to eat less at one sitting than older children and adults and, thus, eat more frequently during the day. When these children were considered separately, the average percentages of total calories per eating occasion (weighted proportionally by the

TABLE 6-2 Percentage of Energy Intake by Eating Occasion, Age, and Gender

| | Calories (kcal) | | | | | |
| | | | 5–10 Years | | 11–13 Years | |
	1 Year	2–4 Years	Males	Females	Males	Females
Breakfast	20	20	22	21	24	22
Lunch	22	27	32	31	30	31
Dinner	22	27	32	31	35	37
Snack	36	26	14	17	11	10

NOTE: After summing the meal percents, the percentage of calories remaining in the day was assigned to snacks.

TABLE 6-3 Proposed Distribution of Calories Across Eating Occasions for All Age Groups

| | | Breakfast | | Lunch | |
Age Group (years)	Total Calories (kcal)	Target Calorie Level (kcal)	% of Total Calories	Target Calorie Level (kcal)	% of Total Calories
1	950	190	20	247	26
2–4	1,300	260	20	338	26
5–10	1,900	418	22	608	32
11–13	1,900	418	22	608	32
14–18	2,400	528	22	768	32
19–59	2,000	440	22	640	32
≥ 60	2,000	440	22	640	32

NOTE: kcal = calories.

years in each of the two youngest age groups) were 20, 26, and 26 percent for breakfast, lunch, and dinner, respectively, leaving 28 percent for snacks. For older children and adults, the corresponding percentages were 22, 31, and 35 percent, leaving 12 percent for snacks.

The committee applied information about the distribution of calories across eating occasions (Table 6-2) to the Estimated Energy Requirement (EER) rounded to the nearest MyPyramid calorie level for each of the child and adult age groups (Table 6-3) to identify target calorie levels for CACFP meals and snacks that are reasonably consistent with current eating patterns. The general formula used is shown in Box 6-2.

Table 6-3 summarizes the committee's recommended calorie targets for each age group for the five possible CACFP eating occasions: breakfast, lunch, supper, and two snacks. For each meal and snack, the table shows both the absolute calorie target and the percentage of total calories. For children ages 5 years and older and adults, the calculated percentages for

Calories (kcal)					
14–18 Years		19–59 Years		≥ 60 Years	
Males	Females	Males	Females	Males	Females
22	22	21	20	24	23
34	35	33	34	33	33
39	39	40	39	41	39
5	4	6	7	2	5

SOURCE: NHANES 2003–2004 for percent of calories at breakfast, lunch, and dinner by those consuming these meals.

Dinner		Snack 1		Snack 2	
Target Caloric Level (kcal)	% of Total Calories	Target Caloric Level (kcal)	% of Total Calories	Target Caloric Level (kcal)	% of Total Calories
247	26	133	14	133	14
338	26	182	14	182	14
608	32	133	7	133	7
608	32	133	7	133	7
768	32	168	7	168	7
640	32	140	7	140	7
640	32	140	7	140	7

BOX 6-2
Formula for Determining Target Calorie
Levels for Meals and Snacks

The general formula used to identify target calorie levels is

Target meal calories =
Mean energy requirement for age group × mean % of calories in meal.

For example, for children ages 2–4 years, the NHANES data indicated that children in this age range obtain an average of 20 percent of total calories from breakfast. Using this information, the target calorie level for breakfast for this age group was calculated as follows:

Breakfast calories = 1,300 calories × 0.2 = 260 calories.

---

some of the eating occasions were adjusted slightly to 32 percent for lunch and supper and 14 percent for snacks. This was done to allow for more calories in snacks and, for reasons of practicality, to make the target calorie levels for lunch and supper the same.

The committee recognizes that some children and adults with limited access to food or with substantially higher calorie needs might benefit from meals or snacks that provide substantially more calories (and nutrients). In the committee's view, however, this situation does not provide the basis for increasing the target calorie levels for CACFP meals and snacks. For children ages 5 years and older and for adults, however, the committee proposed an enhanced snack (see Chapter 7). In addition, family-style meal service, which currently is an option for child care facilities, offers the opportunity to balance the needs of those who need less food (because they are smaller or less hungry) with those who need more. To address the higher needs of vulnerable children and adults, child and adult care programs should use other mechanisms such as referrals to other community nutrition assistance programs (especially including the Supplemental Nutrition Assistance Program) to help ensure that they and their households have access to sufficient food.

Nutrient Targets for Protein, Vitamins, and Minerals

In setting the nutrient targets for CACFP meals and snacks, the committee followed the methodology developed and implemented by the School Meals committee (IOM, 2010). This methodology—referred to as the "Target Median Intake Approach"—was based on the methods recommended for planning daily diets for groups in the report *Dietary Reference Intakes: Applications in Dietary Planning* (IOM, 2003).

Overview of the Target Median Intake Approach

The overall goal of planning intakes for groups of people is to achieve usual daily intakes within the group that meet the requirements of most individuals without being excessive (IOM, 2003). This goal is accomplished by combining information on the group's usual nutrient intakes with information on the group's nutrient requirements (expressed as either an EAR or AI and a Tolerable Upper Intake Level [UL]). The target nutrient intake distribution that is chosen aims to achieve the combined goal of a low predicted prevalence of nutrient inadequacy and a low predicted prevalence of excessive intakes. The median of this intake distribution is the Target Median Intake (TMI). The TMI was the starting point for the committee's calculations to derive the nutrient targets for CACFP meals. The process for setting the initial TMIs for nutrients for children and adults differs depending on whether the nutrient has an EAR or an AI; both processes are described below. TMIs for nutrients are presented in Tables 6-4 and 6-5 for children and adults, respectively.

Setting Targets for Nutrients with an Estimated Average Requirement

Background For most nutrients with an EAR, the current prevalence of inadequacy may be estimated using the EAR cut-point method (IOM, 2006a). If the prevalence of inadequacy is too high, then one goal of the planning process is to reduce the prevalence of inadequacy to an acceptable level. Thus, one of the steps in planning for the nutrient intake of groups is to select the target prevalence of inadequacy. In keeping with the approach used previously by the School Meals committee, this committee set 5 percent rather than the more conservative 2 to 3 percent that has been suggested as an acceptable level of inadequacy (IOM, 2003).

The EARs used to determine the TMIs for children ages 5–10 and 11–13 years are weighted averages of two age groups. The use of weighted averages was necessary because these two age groups span parts of two DRI age groups (4–8 and 9–13 years). The weighting factor was the proportion of the 5-year age span. For example, for the age group 5–10 years, the weighted average was four-sixths (2/3) of the requirement for ages 4–8 years and two-sixths (1/3) of the requirement for ages 9–13 years.

Methodological approach The method recommended in *Dietary Reference Intakes: Applications in Dietary Planning* (IOM, 2003) involves determining the nutrient intake distributions that will result in approximately a 5 percent prevalence of inadequacy. Using this method, the committee shifted each current intake distribution upward or downward until approximately 5 percent of the group's intakes were below the EAR. This method for determining the target distribution assumes that a change in the nutrient content of the daily diet would apply to everyone; thus, the distribution of usual nutrient intakes would shift without changing the shape of the distribution.[1] Under this assumption, the appropriate change in the nutrient intake distribution was calculated as follows:

- The 5th percentile of the intake distribution was positioned at the EAR.
- The new median of the distribution was calculated as the original median plus the difference between the intake at the 5th percentile and the EAR.

If intake at the 5th percentile of the current intake distribution is above the EAR, the new median would be below the current median. *The new median is the TMI for the day.* The same method was used for all vitamins and minerals with an EAR except for iron (see discussion of iron below). For protein, the TMI is expressed in grams per kilogram of body weight (the EAR units for protein). To convert the value to grams of protein per day, it is necessary to assume a body weight for the children in each age-grade group. The committee used median body weights identified in NHANES 2003–2004 (see Chapter 3, Table 3-2) for the midpoint ages in each age group and averaged the weights for males and females. For the youngest children, the committee used median weights for comparable age groups in the report *WIC Food Packages: Time for a Change* (IOM, 2006b).

To illustrate the method, the vitamin C TMI for children ages 2–4 years is used as an example:

1. NHANES data show that vitamin C *intakes* at the 5th percentile are 30 mg per day.
2. The EAR for vitamin C (weighted average) is 16 mg per day.

Therefore, intakes at the 5th percentile exceed the EAR by an average of 14 mg per day, and there is no need to increase intakes. The TMI can be set at 14 mg per day less than the current median intake:

3. Current median intake is 89 mg per day.
4. The TMI is 75 mg per day (89–14).

---

[1] The committee recognizes the weaknesses of this assumption; however, the method provides useful estimates, and a superior alternative method has not been developed.

Setting Targets for Nutrients with an Adequate Intake

Some nutrients have an AI rather than an EAR. Based on guidance from the report *Dietary Reference Intakes: Applications in Dietary Planning* (IOM, 2003), the committee assumed that a low prevalence of inadequacy would result if the median of the usual intake distribution was at least equal to the AI. Thus, for five nutrients with an AI (calcium, potassium, fiber, linoleic acid, and α-linolenic acid), the TMI was set at the AI. As was done with the EARs, weighted averages were used for the AIs for age groups 2–4 and 5–10 years. Although the derivation of the AI differs substantially among these nutrients and among different age-gender groups, the AI is still the most appropriate type of DRI to use to set the TMI.

Sodium The approach used to address sodium did not involve setting a TMI. Instead, the committee agreed to set maximum daily targets for sodium that are based on the age-specific ULs. This decision was made for several reasons. The NHANES (2003–2004) data demonstrated that the AIs for sodium are substantially lower than what children and adults consume, on average. Recognizing that sodium intake in the United States far exceeds the AI and also the UL, the sodium recommendation in the 2005 *Dietary Guidelines for Americans* (HHS/USDA, 2005) is 2.3 g per day—the value of the UL for persons 14 years and older. (The ULs for children younger than 14 years are slightly lower than 2.3 g per day.) Basing the sodium target on the UL rather than the AI is more consistent with achieving meals that are palatable and thus acceptable. For sodium, the goal would be to reduce the median intake to the UL.

Vitamin D A TMI was not set for vitamin D (which has an AI) because of a lack of reliable data on the vitamin D content of foods and on vitamin D intakes. Furthermore, vitamin D sources are highly variable and not under the control of CACFP providers.

Setting the Maximum for Saturated Fat and Cholesterol,
Ranges for Total Fat, and Addressing trans *Fat*

Limiting the intakes of saturated fat, cholesterol, and *trans* fat helps support healthful levels of blood lipids. Avoiding excessive total fat intake also helps control saturated fat intake and helps avoid the intake of excessive calories. On the other hand, moderate intake of healthy fats (unsaturated vegetable oils, soft margarine, nuts, and seeds) helps ensure adequate intake of vitamin E and essential fatty acids, helps support a normal pattern of growth, and may help avoid undesirable changes in blood lipids (HHS/USDA, 2005).

TABLE 6-4 Daily CACFP Target Median Intakes[a] for Children Compar to MyPyramid Food Intake Patterns

Nutrient	TMI for 1 Year	1,000 calories/d MyPyramid Pattern	TMI for 2–4 Years[b]
Protein (g)[d]	27	42	40
Vitamin A (μg RAE)	431	455	462
Vitamin C (mg)	71	73	76
Vitamin E (mg αT)	**6.5**	4.5	**7.1**
Thiamin (mg)	0.82	1.0	0.90
Riboflavin (mg)	1.2	1.5	1.21
Niacin (mg)	10.3	9.7	11.8
Vitamin B_6 (mg)	0.90	1.1	0.98
Folate (μg DFE)	271	306	316
Vitamin B_{12} (μg)	2.7	4.3	2.8
Iron (mg)	7.4	7.6	8.5
Magnesium (mg)	131	180	148
Zinc (mg)	5.4	6.6	6.3
Calcium (mg)	500	782	600
Phosphorus (mg)	780	905	836
Potassium (mg)	**3,000**	1,988	**3,267**
Sodium (mg)[f]	1,500	869	1,633
Linoleic acid (g)	7.0	9.3	8.0
α-linolenic acid (g)	0.70	0.9	0.77
Fiber (g)	**19.0**	13.0	**21.0**

NOTE: The goal is to offer diets that provide at least the amount of nutrient listed in the TMI column for each age group. The MyPyramid columns show the amount of each nutrient that the pattern would provide given the target calorie level for the age group. αT = α-tocopherol; d = day; DFE = dietary folate equivalent; g = gram; kg = kilogram; μg = microgram; mg = milligram; RAE = retinol activity equivalent; TMI = Target Median Intake.

[a]TMIs are calculated based on a 5% prevalence of inadequacy for nutrients with an EAR. Those shown in bold font are higher than the amounts provided by the MyPyramid pattern.

[b]TMIs shown for the 2–4-year-old and 5–10-year-old age groups are calculated using weighted averages of the EARs and AIs for two DRI age groups.

[c]The 1,300-calories-per-day pattern is an average of the 1,200- and 1,400-calorie patterns; the 1,900-calories-per-day pattern is an average of the 1,800- and 2,000-calorie patterns.

The committee relied on recommendations from 2005 *Dietary Guidelines* (HHS/USDA, 2005) to set a target maximum intake for saturated fat and cholesterol (substances in food that are not essential nutrients) and ranges of intake for total fat (IOM, 2002/2005). In particular, the *Dietary Guidelines* recommends a fat intake of 25 to 35 percent of total calories, less than 10 percent of calories from saturated fatty acids (which are abundant in the fat in dairy products and meat), and a maximum of 300 mg of cholesterol per day for all individuals over the age of 2 years (HHS/USDA,

1,300 calories/d MyPyramid Pattern[c]	TMI for 5–13 Years[b]	1,900 calories/d MyPyramid Pattern[c]	TMI for 14–18 Years	2,400 calories/d MyPyramid Pattern
59	**92**	89	97	105
639	670	1,032	847	1,126
96	89	143	116	163
5.9	**10.3**	9.1	**16.4**	10.7
1.4	1.2	2.0	1.7	2.4
1.9	1.6	2.8	2.0	3.1
15.0	15.3	21.4	19.8	27.3
1.6	1.4	2.4	1.8	2.9
445	442	682	631	822
5.5	3.7	8.2	4.6	9.2
11.6	10.5[e]	17.3	18.6	21.5
244	254	372	440	440
9.4	10.0	14.0	12.5	16.7
866	1,198	1,309	**1,504**	1,388
1,142	1,287	1,716	1,713	1,901
2,568	**4,596**	3,914	**5,438**	4,523
1,227	2,265	1,750	2,025	2,136
11.6	11.4	16.8	14.1	20.9
1.1	1.1	1.7	1.4	2.0
19.5	29.0	30.0	33.5	37.0

[d]Assumes body weights of 11.6 kg for children age 1 year, 16.1 kg for children age 2 years, 30.6 kg for males ages 5–10 years, 31.2 kg for females ages 5–10 years, 54.3 kg for males ages 11–13 years, 53.6 kg for females ages 11–13 years, 73.0 kg for males ages 14–18 years, and 63.2 kg for females ages 14–18 years (NHANES 2003–2004).

[e]Methods used to calculate iron values for females 11–13 years old are described in Chapter 4.

[f]Sodium TMIs are based on the Tolerable Upper Intake Levels (UL).

SOURCE: Nutrient values in columns representing the MyPyramid patterns are from Britten et al., 2006.

2005). The committee used these values as the basis for the fat targets for CACFP meals and snacks. For children 1 year of age, a more liberal allowance (30 to 40 percent of total calories) was used for total fat. The goal was to keep saturated fat and cholesterol as low as practical. These targets are consistent with the goals defined for this age group in *Dietary Reference Intakes* (IOM, 2002/2005). The committee considered the *Dietary Guidelines* plus supplementary information to address whether it would be possible to set a target maximum for *trans* fat (see Box 6-3).

TABLE 6-5 Daily Target Median Intakes[a] for Adults Compared to MyPyramid Food Intake Patterns

Nutrient	TMI for ≥ 19 Years[c]	2,000 calories/d MyPyramid pattern
Protein (g)[b]	**104**	91
Vitamin A (μg RAE)	988	1,052
Vitamin C (mg)	135	155
Vitamin E (mg αT)	**18.5**	9.5
Thiamin (mg)	1.8	2.0
Riboflavin (mg)	2.1	2.8
Niacin (mg)	**22.6**	21.9
Vitamin B$_6$ (mg)	**2.5**	2.4
Folate (μg DFE)	647	695
Vitamin B$_{12}$ (μg)	5.0	8.3
Iron (mg)	12.6	17.5
Magnesium (mg)	**451**	380
Zinc (mg)	13.6	14.3
Calcium (mg)	**1,519**	1,316
Phosphorus (mg)	1,231	1,740
Potassium (mg)	**5,950**	4,044
Sodium (mg)[d]	**1,873**	1,779
Linoleic acid (g)	13.9	17.7
α-linolenic acid (g)	1.5	1.7
Fiber (g)	29.0	31.0

NOTE: The goal is to offer diets that provide at least the amount of nutrient listed in the TMI column for each age group. The MyPyramid columns show the amount of each nutrient that the pattern would provide given the target calorie level for the age group. αT = α-tocopherol; d = day; DFE = dietary folate equivalent; g = gram; kg = kilogram; μg = microgram; mg = milligram; RAE = retinol activity equivalent; TMI = Target Median Intake.

[a]TMIs are calculated based on a 5% prevalence of inadequacy for nutrients with an EAR. Those shown in bold font are higher than the amounts provided by the MyPyramid pattern.

[b]Assumes body weights of 88.0 for males ages 19–59 years, 75.3 kg for females ages 19–59 years, 87.3 kg for males ages ≥ 60 years, and 73.0 kg for females ages ≥ 60 years (NHANES 2003–2004).

[c]These TMIs shown for the 19–59-year-old age group are calculated using weighted averages of the EARs or AIs for multiple DRI age groups.

[d]Sodium TMIs are based on the Tolerable Upper Intake Levels (UL).

SOURCE: Nutrient values in columns representing the MyPyramid patterns are from Britten et al., 2006.

Calculating Target Median Intakes for CACFP Age Groups

To incorporate the TMI concept into the setting of the nutrient targets for CACFP meals and snacks, the committee first addressed the fact that, for some age groups, nutrient needs differ substantially for males and females. The committee aimed to calculate targets for total daily intake that would best reflect these differences in nutrient needs. The committee used the simple nutrient density approach, as implemented by the School Meals

---

BOX 6-3
***trans* Fats**

The *Dietary Guidelines for Americans* (HHS/USDA, 2005) recommends that *trans* fat intake be kept as low as possible, but it does not specify a maximum level of intake. In turn, no data exist on which to base a maximum level for *trans* fat in CACFP meals and snacks, even though the goal is essentially zero grams. Nonetheless, a practical method can be used to keep the *trans* fat content of CACFP meals to a minimum. In particular, this is achievable by specifying that, for any food included on the menu, zero grams of *trans* fat per serving would be the maximum amount of *trans* fat listed on the nutrition label. This method is not always applicable because some products, such as bakery items produced by manufacturers who qualify as small businesses, are exempted from nutrition labeling, and thus the *trans* fat content of the product may not be specified. The committee notes that foods labeled as containing zero grams of *trans* fat may actually contain a small amount (< 0.5 grams) of *trans* fat per serving.

---

committee to combine the TMIs by gender for each age group.[2,3] Using this approach for males and females separately within each of the age groups beginning at 5 years, the committee calculated the nutrient density (the ratio of the gender-specific TMI to the gender-specific EER) that is shown in Table 6-2. It then multiplied the *higher density* times the mean EER for the age group to obtain the candidate TMI. This approach was not necessary for children under 5 years of age because males and females have similar intakes and requirements.

Comparing Daily CACFP Target Median Intakes with MyPyramid Food Patterns

Because the MyPyramid food patterns were designed to meet the 2005 *Dietary Guidelines* (HHS/USDA, 2005), potentially they could provide a sound basis for recommended meal and snack patterns for CACFP. To test this, the committee compared the daily CACFP TMIs for each age group with the nutrient content of the MyPyramid food pattern for the corresponding daily calorie target, as also shown in Tables 6-4 and 6-5. For

---

[2]The term *nutrient density* has been used in different ways in the literature. The usage presented here is the one presented in *Dietary Reference Intakes: Applications in Dietary Planning* (IOM, 2003). This usage applies to setting a target for daily intake of each nutrient relative to daily calorie needs.

[3]See the report *School Meals: Building Blocks for Healthy Children* (IOM, 2010, pp. 80–81) for a discussion of the limitations of the nutrient density approach and other alternatives that were considered but ultimately rejected by the School Meals committee.

almost all nutrients, the CACFP TMI value was lower than the amount that would be obtained by following the MyPyramid pattern for the calorie level set for each age group. That is, providing meals that are based on the MyPyramid pattern provides nutrients in amounts that are close to or exceed the nutrient targets while helping achieve alignment with the *Dietary Guidelines*.

For most age groups of children, vitamin E and potassium are the only nutrients that would be provided by the MyPyramid pattern in amounts below the CACFP TMI. For age groups 1 and 2–4 years, fiber amounts would also be somewhat below the CACFP TMI. For the 14–18-year age group, calcium amounts would also be lower than the CACFP TMI.

The comparison is slightly less favorable for the adults (see Table 6-5). In particular, the MyPyramid pattern provides protein, vitamin E, magnesium, calcium, and potassium in amounts that are substantially below the CACFP TMI. When the totality of nutrients were considered, however, the committee concluded that following a meal pattern based on MyPyramid would provide adequate nutrient levels to adult CACFP participants for the meals and snacks served.

Converting Daily CACFP Target Median Intakes to Meal and Snack Nutrient Targets

The CACFP TMIs (Tables 6-4 and 6-5) are for total daily intake. However, each CACFP meal and snack provides only a portion of the day's intake. As described earlier in this chapter, the committee set targets for the percentage of total calories to be provided by the CACFP meals and snacks (see Table 6-3). In developing recommendations for the calorie targets for CACFP meals and snacks, the committee multiplied the CACFP TMIs by the percentages in Table 6-3 to obtain nutrient targets for the meals. For example, the targets for breakfast for the 2–4-year age group represent 20 percent of the respective CACFP TMIs, and the targets for lunch for the same age group represent 26 percent. Daily nutrient targets averaged over a 5-day week for CACFP meals and snacks appear in Appendix Tables J-1 through J-3. The committee multiplied the sodium UL by the calorie percentages in Table 6-3 to obtain preliminary maximum intakes rather than nutrient targets.

The committee recognizes that the target nutrient intake distribution would be achieved only if participants' intakes from CACFP meals and snacks were accompanied by similar changes in the nutrient intakes from foods consumed outside the program. That is, the recommended amounts of nutrients from the CACFP meals and snacks would need to be consumed, and comparable intakes would have to be sustained across the full day's intake, in order to meet the CACFP TMI and achieve no greater than 5 percent prevalence of inadequacy. Nonetheless, it is desirable to set nutrient targets for CACFP meals and snacks to provide a scientific basis for the Meal Requirements and also to serve as a model for the meals and snacks served in other child and adult care settings. Even if only an afterschool snack is served by CACFP, the types and amounts of the foods may promote the desire for, and acceptance of, a higher quality diet throughout the rest of the day.

Considering the Tolerable Upper Intake Level in Setting Nutrient Targets

The committee examined the possibility that, for some nutrients, the prevalence of intakes above the UL would be undesirably high if the CACFP TMIs were achieved for the full day's intake. Using NHANES (2003–2004) data, an *adjusted* intake at the 95th percentile was calculated assuming that the median intake of a nutrient changed to be equal to the CACFP TMI and that the whole distribution (including the 95th percentile) would change by the same amount. For these analyses, intakes of 5–10-year-olds were not combined with those of 11–13-year-olds, nor were intakes of younger (19–59 years) and older (≥ 60 years) adults; calculations were performed separately for males and females within each age group. This same method was used for nutrients with an EAR and for nutrients with an AI.

For each age group, the adjusted intake at the 95th percentile was compared to the UL, if any. (Magnesium was excluded because the UL is only for pharmacological agents. The UL does not apply to magnesium in foods [IOM, 1997].) For children ages 5–10 years, the UL for the younger DRI age group (6–8 years)—the most conservative value—was used. For several nutrients, the ULs are considerably lower for children ages 8 years or younger than for older children.

The results are shown in Tables 6-6 and 6-7. For each age group, there were some nutrients with the adjusted 95th percentile of intakes above the UL, meaning that at least 5 percent of CACFP participants would have intakes above the UL if the median intake was at the CACFP TMI, as follows:

- 1-year-olds: vitamin A, niacin, folate, zinc, and sodium
- 2–4-year-olds: vitamin A, niacin, folate, zinc, and sodium
- 5–10-year-olds: vitamin A, niacin, folate, zinc, and sodium for males and females
- 11–13-year-olds: niacin, folate, and sodium for males and females
- 14–18-year-olds: niacin, folate, and sodium for males and females
- 19–59-year-olds: folate and sodium for males and females; niacin for males
- 60-year-olds and older: sodium for males and females; niacin and folate for males

TABLE 6-6 Children: Tolerable Upper Intake Level (UL) for Nutrients with a UL,* Reported Intakes,**[a] and Predicted Adjusted Intakes at the 95th Percentile, and Adjusted Intakes as a Percentage of the UL, by Age-Gender Group

	1 Year				2–4 Years			
	Males and Females				Males and Females			
Nutrient (unit)	UL[b]	Intake at 95th	Adj. Intake at 95th	Adj. Intake as % of UL	UL[b]	Intake at 95th	Adj. Intake at 95th	Adj. Intake as % of UL
Vitamin A (µg RAE/d)	600	883	831	138	600	878	840	140
Vitamin C (mg/d)	400	212	190	48	400	207	194	48
Vitamin E (mg αT/d)	200	6.5	9.4	5	200	6.8	9.9	5
Niacin (mg/d)	10.0	21.4	18.6	186	10.0	24.4	21.5	215
Vitamin B_6 (mg/d)	30.0	2.2	1.8	6	30.0	2.4	2.0	7
Folate (µg DFE/d)	300	637	550	183	300	735	655	218
Iron (mg/d)	40.0	17.9	15.0	38	40.0	19.4	16.5	41
Magnesium (mg/d)	65	278	225	346	65	286	243	375
Zinc (mg/d)	7.0	12.4	9.9	142	7.0	13.7	11.5	164
Calcium (mg/d)	2,500	1,590	1,135	45	2,500	1,591	1,224	49
Phosphorus (mg/d)	3,000	1,603	1,334	44	3,000	1,623	1,375	46
Sodium (mg/d)	1,500	3,233	2,731	182	1,500	3,629	3,050	203

	Males				Females			
	5–10 Years							
Vitamin A (µg RAE/d)	900	909	1,016	113	900	863	996	111
Vitamin C (mg/d)	650	179	191	29	650	175	187	29
Vitamin E (mg αT/d)	300	8.8	13.9	5	300	8.0	13.3	4
Niacin (mg/d)	15.0	31.9	26.9	179	15.0	28.0	24.2	161
Vitamin B_6 (mg/d)	40.0	2.6	2.4	6	40.0	2.4	2.3	6
Folate (µg DFE/d)	400	968	874	218	400	828	760	190
Iron (mg/d)	40.0	22.8	18.4	46	40.0	20.7	17.3	43
Magnesium (mg/d)	110	329	362	329	110	297	342	311
Zinc (mg/d)	12.0	18.3	17.4	145	12.0	15.0	14.9	124
Calcium (mg/d)	2,500	1,620	1,822	73	2,500	1,557	1,816	73
Phosphorus (mg/d)	3,000	1,836	1,873	62	3,000	1,690	1,816	61
Sodium (mg/d)	1,900	4,553	3,772	199	1,900	4,132	3,576	188

TABLE 6-6 Continued

	Males				Females		
		11–13 Years					
Nutrient (unit)	UL[b]	Intake at 95th	Adj. Intake at 95th	Adj. Intake as % of UL	UL[b]	Intake at 95th	Adj. Intake at 95th	Adj. Intake as % of UL
Vitamin A (µg RAE/d)	1,700	1,005	1,114	66	1,700	802	978	58
Vitamin C (mg/d)	1,200	157	169	14	1,200	151	163	14
Vitamin E (mg αT/d)	600	10.3	14.1	2	600	8.9	13.7	2
Niacin (mg/d)	20.0	35.8	28.0	140	20.0	28.9	24.9	125
Vitamin B$_6$ (mg/d)	60	2.8	2.4	4	60	2.3	2.2	4
Folate (µg DFE/d)	600	1,046	892	149	600	763	702	117
Iron (mg/d)	40.0	24.8	18.6	47	40.0	20.2	17.0	42
Magnesium (mg/d)	350	368	376	107	350	300	347	99
Zinc (mg/d)	23.0	21.3	18.4	80	23.0	14.1	14.4	63
Calcium (mg/d)	2,500	1,704	1,831	73	2,500	1,438	1,759	70
Phosphorus (mg/d)	4,000	1,987	1,880	47	4,000	1,658	1,812	45
Sodium (mg/d)	2,200	5,006	3,747	170	2,200	4,384	3,124	142

	Males				Females		
		14–18 Years					
Vitamin A (µg RAE/d)	2,800	1,141	1,428	51	2,800	869	1,262	45
Vitamin C (mg/d)	1,800	204	240	13	1,800	161	211	12
Vitamin E (mg αT/d)	800	12.8	22.7	3	800	9.5	20.3	3
Niacin (mg/d)	30.0	41.5	34.7	116	30.0	28.0	28.1	94
Vitamin B$_6$ (mg/d)	80	3.5	3.3	4	80	2.4	2.7	3
Folate (µg DFE/d)	800	1,225	1,244	155	800	857	1,008	126
Iron (mg/d)	45.0	31.7	32.2	72	45.0	21.2	26.4	59
Magnesium (mg/d)	350	473	638	182	350	329	561	160
Zinc (mg/d)	34.0	22.9	21.1	62	34.0	15.5	18.0	53
Calcium (mg/d)	2,500	2,103	2,467	99	2,500	1,385	2,074	83
Phosphorus (mg/d)	4,000	2,487	2,653	66	4,000	1,702	2,277	57
Sodium (mg/d)	2,300	6,212	4,287	186	2,300	4,255	3,270	142

NOTES: αT = α-tocopherol; d = day; DFE = dietary folate equivalent; g = gram; kg = kilogram; µg = microgram; mg = milligram; RAE = retinol activity equivalent. Bold font indicates intake values above the UL.

[a]Intakes exclude contributions from nutrient supplements.

[b]The UL listed is the lowest UL value within the age-gender group.

SOURCES: *IOM, 2006a; **NHANES 2003–2004.

TABLE 6-7 Adults: Tolerable Upper Intake Level (UL) for Nutrients with a UL,* Reported Intakes,**[a] and Predicted Adjusted Intakes at the 95th Percentile, and Adjusted Intakes as a Percentage of the UL, by Age-Gender Group

		Males				Females		
					19–59 Years			
Nutrient (unit)	UL[b]	Intake at 95th	Adj. Intake at 95th	Adj. Intake as % of UL	UL[b]	Intake at 95th	Adj. Intake at 95th	Adj. Intake as % of UL
Vitamin A (µg RAE/d)	3,000	1,268	1,651	55	3,000	987	1,498	50
Vitamin C (mg/d)	2,000	209	263	13	2,000	187	250	13
Vitamin E (mg αT/d)	1,000	13.8	24.5	2	1,000	10.9	23.2	2
Niacin (mg/d)	35.0	**46.7**	39.1	112	35.0	30.9	33.8	96
Vitamin B₆ (mg/d)	100	3.6	3.9	4	100	2.7	3.6	4
Folate (µg DFE/d)	1,000	**1,067**	1,108	111	1,000	838	1,035	103
Iron (mg/d)	45.0	30.4	24.8	55	45.0	21.6	21.1	47
Magnesium (mg/d)	350	**520**	647	185	350	**381**	605	173
Zinc (mg/d)	40.0	23.3	22.3	56	40.0	16.5	20.3	51
Calcium (mg/d)	2,500	1,866	2,383	95	2,500	1,390	2,151	86
Phosphorus (mg/d)	4,000	2,475	2,074	52	4,000	1,807	1,910	48
Sodium (mg/d)	2,300	**6,534**	4,126	179	2,300	**4,570**	3,398	148
					≥ 60 Years			
Vitamin A (µg RAE/d)	3,000	1,497	1,894	63	3,000	1,027	1,470	49
Vitamin C (mg/d)	2,000	177	238	12	2,000	163	229	11
Vitamin E (mg αT/d)	1,000	13.8	25.9	3	1,000	10.4	23.4	2
Niacin (mg/d)	35.0	**37.8**	36.5	104	35.0	29.4	22.6	65
Vitamin B₆ (mg/d)	100	3.2	3.8	4	100	2.5	3.5	4
Folate (µg DFE/d)	1,000	950	1,080	108	1,000	749	983	98
Iron (mg/d)	45.0	27.4	24.2	54	45.0	20.3	20.7	46
Magnesium (mg/d)	350	**447**	618	177	350	**356**	584	167
Zinc (mg/d)	40.0	19.6	21.7	54	40.0	15.1	20.1	50
Calcium (mg/d)	2,500	1,478	2,200	88	2,500	1,260	2,125	85
Phosphorus (mg/d)	3,000	2,031	1,990	66	3,000	1,552	1,797	60
Sodium (mg/d)	2,300	**5,293**	3,917	170	2,300	**3,956**	3,274	142

NOTES: αT = α-tocopherol; d = day; DFE = dietary folate equivalent; g = gram; kg = kilogram; µg = microgram; mg = milligram; RAE = retinol activity equivalent. Bold font indicates intake values above the UL.

[a]Intakes exclude contributions from nutrient supplements.

[b]The UL listed is the lowest UL value within the age-gender group.

SOURCES: *IOM, 2006a; **NHANES 2003–2004.

It is worth noting that, in most of these cases, current intakes at the 95th percentile also exceed the UL. As would be expected, at the 95th percentile of intake, all values for sodium are well above the UL. For most nutrients, intakes above the UL are not likely to be a concern. This is largely because the ULs only apply to certain forms or sources of nutrients, whereas the intake estimates are for the total diet. For example, the vitamin A UL applies only to preformed retinol, and the niacin and folate ULs apply only to these nutrients in fortified foods and supplements. These issues are discussed in more detail in the *School Meals* report (IOM, 2010).

DEVELOPING MEAL REQUIREMENTS

The Meal Requirements provide standards for CACFP meals and snacks that serve two purposes: (1) providing patterns and specifications for menus that are consistent with the *Dietary Guidelines* and the nutrient targets, and (2) identifying what qualifies as a meal that is eligible for federal financial reimbursement. The following discussion describes the iterative processes (see Figure 6-1) used to develop recommendations for the Meal Requirements. The committee's final recommendations for CACFP Meal Requirements are presented in Chapter 7.

The Approach

The process used in developing recommended Meal Requirements built on the approach used by the School Meals committee. The approach uses MyPyramid food intake patterns to provide a basis for planning menus that are consistent with the *Dietary Guidelines* and that provide nutrients in amounts that equal or exceed the CACFP TMIs, with two exceptions— vitamin E and potassium. The MyPyramid patterns specify amounts of foods from six major food groups and seven food subgroups—a larger number of food groups than currently used for planning CACFP meals and snacks[4] but a number judged workable by the committee.

Developing Meal Patterns

The process of developing meal patterns for individuals, ages 2 years and older, included (1) calculations to determine amounts that would be consistent with MyPyramid food patterns for specified calorie levels and (2) the evaluation of the patterns in terms of nutrient content, cost, and acceptability. These steps are described below. The approach used for infants

---

[4]Existing rules specify four food groups: vegetable/fruit, grain/bread, meat/meat alternate, and fluid milk.

and children younger than 2 years appears in the later section "Developing Meal Patterns for Infants."

Calculation of Meal Patterns

The MyPyramid food patterns at selected calorie levels were used as the basis to calculate the 5-day amounts of each food group to be served in CACFP. Daily amounts are provided for the major food groups. Therefore, each amount was multiplied by five to calculate the serving sizes over 5 days within the CACFP program. However, because the amounts for the vegetable subgroups in the MyPyramid patterns are provided for a 7-day week, each weekly amount was multiplied by 5/7 to achieve the correct serving size for 5 days in a CACFP meal pattern. For example, in the 1,800-calorie MyPyramid pattern, 3 cups of dark green vegetables should be served weekly (over 7 days). To determine the amount of these vegetables to be served over 5 days, 3 cups was multiplied by 5/7, which equals 2.1 cups of dark green vegetables. Rounding, which is necessary for a practical pattern, occurred at a later step in the process.

The percentage of calories assigned by the committee for each eating occasion was then applied to the 5-day pattern for every food group and subgroup to determine the distribution of food groups for breakfast, lunch and supper, and snacks. This approach kept the food group amounts proportional to the number of calories specified for the meal.

The committee adapted a set of menu development spreadsheets that had been developed by the School Meals committee (IOM, 2010) and used these to test, in an iterative fashion, possible meal patterns against the nutrient targets presented in Tables 6-4 and 6-5. (For a description of the approach and methodology see IOM [2010].) Adjustments to the food groups and serving sizes at each eating occasion were made when necessary to develop a more practical menu pattern.

Writing Menus and Testing Meal Patterns

In the process of developing the meal patterns, the writing of menus based on initial patterns posed practical problems. This led to some adjustment of the patterns. The menu development spreadsheets provided basic information on how the pattern adjustments affected the nutrient content. The methods used for estimating nutrient contents are described in Appendix G. The menus that are based on the recommended patterns appear in Appendix K. Early estimates of the nutrient content of menus reinforced the need to recommend specifications for the types of food items that belong to the five meal components. Information about cost appears in Chapter 8.

Developing Meal Patterns for Infants

For infants and children under 2 years of age, the committee referred to the report *WIC Food Packages* (IOM, 2006b) for food group priorities and nutrient priorities and summarized them in Chapter 4 of this report. The development of meal patterns for the two youngest age groups (0–5 months and 6–11 months) relied primarily on (1) the dietary guidance from the American Academy of Pediatrics (AAP) as presented in Chapter 3, (2) the recommendations for infant food packages in the report *WIC Food Packages: Time for a Change* (IOM, 2006b, Table 6-6), and (3) the specifications for infant foods in that report (IOM, 2006b, Appendix B, Table B-1). The development of meal patterns for 1-year-old children relied on guidance from the AAP, the WIC child food packages (IOM, 2006b, Table 6-4), and MyPyramid (USDA, 2010).

SUMMARY

The process for developing revised Meal Requirements for the CACFP began with the development of criteria and involved five complex steps including the setting of parameters, assessment of dietary intake, setting of nutrient targets, developing meal patterns and food specifications, and using the criteria to iteratively evaluate and finalize the Meal Requirement recommendations. The next chapter presents the committee's recommendations for meal patterns and food specifications.

REFERENCES

Britten, P., K. Marcoe, S. Yamini, and C. Davis. 2006. Development of food intake patterns for the MyPyramid Food Guidance System. *Journal of Nutrition Education and Behavior* 38(6 Suppl):S78–S92.

HHS/USDA (U.S. Department of Health and Human Services/U.S. Department of Agriculture). 2005. *Dietary Guidelines for Americans*, 6th ed. Washington, DC: U.S. Government Printing Office. http://www.health.gov/DietaryGuidelines/dga2005/document/ (accessed July 23, 2008).

IOM (Institute of Medicine). 1997. *Dietary Reference Intakes for Calcium, Phosphorus, Magnesium, Vitamin D, and Fluoride*. Washington, DC: National Academy Press.

IOM. 1998. *Dietary Reference Intakes for Thiamin, Riboflavin, Niacin, Vitamin B_6, Folate, Vitamin B_{12}, Pantothenic Acid, Biotin, and Choline*. Washington, DC: National Academy Press.

IOM. 2000. *Dietary Reference Intakes for Vitamin C, Vitamin E, Selenium, and Carotenoids*. Washington, DC: National Academy Press.

IOM. 2001. *Dietary Reference Intakes for Vitamin A, Vitamin K, Arsenic, Boron, Chromium, Copper, Iodine, Iron, Manganese, Molybdenum, Nickel, Silicon, Vanadium, and Zinc*. Washington, DC: National Academy Press.

IOM. 2002/2005. *Dietary Reference Intakes for Energy, Carbohydrate, Fiber, Fat, Fatty Acids, Cholesterol, Protein, and Amino Acids*. Washington, DC: The National Academies Press.

IOM. 2003. *Dietary Reference Intakes: Applications in Dietary Planning*. Washington, DC: The National Academies Press.

IOM. 2005. *Dietary Reference Intakes for Water, Potassium, Sodium, Chloride, and Sulfate*. Washington, DC: The National Academies Press.

IOM. 2006a. *Dietary Reference Intakes: The Essential Guide to Nutrient Requirements*. Washington, DC: The National Academies Press.

IOM. 2006b. *WIC Food Packages: Time for a Change*. Washington, DC: The National Academies Press.

IOM. 2010. *School Meals: Building Blocks for Healthy Children*. Washington, DC: The National Academies Press.

7

Recommendations for Meal Requirements

This chapter presents recommendations for revised Meal Requirements for the Child and Adult Care Food Program (CACFP). As structured by the committee, the revised Meal Requirements encompass two distinct elements: meal patterns and food specifications. This chapter begins with three Meal Requirement recommendations, which cover (1) recommended meal patterns for infants up to 1 year of age, (2) recommended meal patterns for children ages 1 year or older and adults, and (3) an option for an enhanced afternoon snack. Then the chapter provides detailed information about recommended meal patterns for the different age groups and the proposed food specifications.

RECOMMENDED MEAL REQUIREMENTS

In order to bring the Meal Requirements into alignment with the best available dietary guidance and to improve consistency with the requirements of other U.S. Department of Agriculture (USDA) food programs, the committee developed the following three recommendations for the Food and Nutrition Service of USDA. The meal pattern tables that are identified as part of the recommendations appear in the section "Recommended Meal and Snack Patterns" and the table of food specifications appears in the section "Food Specifications."

Improve Nutritional Quality of CACFP Meals and Snacks over Time and in Alignment with Dietary Guidance

Meal Requirement Recommendation 1: **USDA should adopt the recommended Meal Requirements for healthy infants up to 1 year of age** (shown in Tables 7-1 and 7-8). Key elements of this recommendation are

- the provision of only breast milk or formula for infants under 6 months of age;
- the gradual introduction of baby meats, cereals, fruits, and vegetables beginning at age 6 months; and
- the omission of fruit juice of any type before the age of 1 year.

In addition, for infants 6–11 months of age, when solid foods are introduced, it is recommended to introduce meat as the preferred first solid food to help ensure an iron source for breastfed infants (AAP, 2009; Krebs et al., 2006). Practices that promote breastfeeding should be encouraged.

Meal Requirement Recommendation 2: **For all children age 1 year and older and for adults, USDA should adopt Meal Requirements that increase the variety of fruits and vegetables, increase the proportion of whole grains, and decrease the content of solid fats, added sugars, *trans* fats, and sodium** (shown in Tables 7-2 through 7-8). Key elements of this recommendation follow:

- One fruit and two vegetables are to be served at each lunch and supper meal. Over the course of a 5-day week, different types of vegetables are to be served at each lunch and supper, as follows: dark green vegetables at least twice per week, orange vegetables at least twice/week,[1] legumes at least once/week, starchy vegetables no more than twice per week, and other vegetables at least three times per week. Appendix Table H-1 lists vegetables in each vegetable subgroup. Serving sizes are tailored to the age group's nutritional needs.
- Fruit rather than fruit juice is to be served at most meals; unsweetened 100 percent juice is allowed only once per day in a serving size tailored to the age group's needs.
- Over the course of the week and day, at least half of the grains/

---

[1]The 2010 Report from the Dietary Guidelines Advisory Committee (available at: http://www.cnpp.usda.gov/DGAs2010-DGACReport.htm [accessed February 10, 2011]) recommends that tomatoes be moved from the other vegetables group to a new group, red/orange vegetables. If incorporated into the *Dietary Guidelines for Americans*, this change will require a minor adjustment to the CACFP weekly vegetable servings to match the new recommendations.

breads served in meals and snacks must be whole grain-rich, meeting the definition given in the table of proposed food specifications (Table 7-8). Other grain/bread must be enriched. Providers are encouraged to gradually increase the proportion of grain foods that are whole grain-rich to well above half of the grain foods and to include 100 percent whole grain foods often.

- Each morning and afternoon snack will provide two different food components in a serving size tailored to the age group's needs; over the course of a 5-day week, the food components provided will include two servings of fruit, one serving of an orange vegetable, one serving of a non-starchy vegetable, two servings of grain/bread, two servings of lean meat or meat alternate, and two servings of low-fat or nonfat milk.

- The amounts of solid fats, added sugars, *trans* fats, and sodium are to be limited in all meals and snacks. For example, milk and yogurt must be low-fat or nonfat for those ages 2 years or older (whole milk for 1-year old children), meats must be lean, fruits and juices must be free of added sugars, foods with nutritional labels must be labeled as containing zero grams of *trans* fat, and foods high in added sugars and/or sodium are to be served infrequently, if at all. Table 7-8 provides guidance.

Incorporating these elements into the Meal Requirements will help ensure the nutritional quality of the meals over time and improve their alignment with the *Dietary Guidelines*.

Each of the vegetable subgroups makes different nutrient contributions. Compared with the common practice of offering only a few kinds of vegetables over the course of weeks, offering varied selections from the combination of vegetable subgroups each week improves the nutritional quality of the diet and alignment with current dietary guidance. The snack pattern also calls for variety to help ensure nutritional quality over time.

Similarly, increased variety was a key component of the Institute of Medicine's recommended revisions of the *WIC Food Packages* (IOM, 2006) and of the *Dietary Guidelines*. For adults, the recommended meal patterns are more consistent with guidance in the publication *Nutrition Service Providers Guide for Older Adults* (HHS/AoA, 2006). In addition, the U.S. Department of Health and Human Services (HHS) Administration on Aging (AoA) (2006), in its *Nutrition Services Providers Guide for Older Adults*, aligns menus for the Older Americans Nutrition Program (commonly called Meals On Wheels) with the *Dietary Guidelines*, separates fruits and vegetables and increases their servings per meal, and recommends averaging menus over a week. It also requires computer analysis of the weekly menus to assess nutrient content in relation to the Dietary Reference Intakes (DRIs) for older adults (HHS/AoA, 2006).

Provide an Enhanced Snack Option for Adults and Children over 5 Years of Age

Meal Requirement Recommendation 3: **USDA should give CACFP providers the option of serving one enhanced snack in the afternoon in place of a smaller snack in both the morning and the afternoon** (shown in Table 7-6). The enhanced snack option would be particularly appropriate for at-risk children in afterschool programs and for older adults because their access to nutritious foods may be limited at home. The enhanced snack would have the same requirements as two of the smaller snacks. Providers would specify in advance which snack option they were choosing and would serve the same type of snack to all participants in their care. The current CACFP monitoring and reimbursement structure would need to be modified to allow for this new option.

RECOMMENDED MEAL AND SNACK PATTERNS

The meal and snack patterns developed by the committee are essential parts of the recommended Meal Requirements. The tables that are presented below show, by eating occasion and age group, the types and amounts of food components that are to be offered. Footnotes in the tables refer the reader to the proposed food specifications. Those specifications are key elements of the Meal Requirements and appear later in this chapter.

Infants

The recommended meal and snack patterns for infants, shown in Table 7-1, increase the consistency of CACFP infant meals with recommendations made by the American Academy of Pediatrics (AAP) (see Table 3-1 in Chapter 3) and also with the Institute of Medicine's recommended revisions for the Supplemental Nutrition Program for Women, Infants, and Children (WIC) food packages for infants (IOM, 2006).

Children and Adults

For children and adults, the recommended weekly meal and snack patterns covered below align CACFP meals and snacks with dietary guidance. For 1-year-old children, the patterns are aligned with recommendations from the AAP and the DRIs. For those ages 2 years and older, the patterns are consistent with the *Dietary Guidelines* and the DRIs. For all the age

TABLE 7-1 Recommended Daily Meal and Snack Patterns for Infants

Infant Age	Meal	Breast Milk/ Infant Formula[a]	Meats, Vegetables, Fruits, and Infant Cereals (Complementary Foods)[a,b]
0–5 months	All feedings	4–6 oz breast milk or infant formula per feeding[c]	No solid foods
6–11 months	Breakfast (meal 1)	6–8 oz breast milk or formula[c]	1–4 T meat, fish, poultry, or egg yolk OR 1–4 T infant cereal[d] PLUS 1–2 T vegetable OR 1–2 T fruit[d]
	Lunch/supper (meals 2 and 3)	6–8 oz breast milk or formula[c]	1–4 T meat, fish, poultry or egg yolk OR 1–4 T infant cereal[d] PLUS 1–2 T vegetable OR 1–2 T fruit[e]
	Snack	2–4 oz breast milk or formula[c]	1–2 T vegetable OR 1–2 T fruit[e] PLUS ½ slice of bread OR 2 crackers

NOTES: Do not serve any type of milk, foods mixed with milk (such as milk with cereal, milk in mashed potatoes), or milk-based products (yogurt, milk, cottage cheese) until 1 year of age. Begin transitioning to cow milk at 1 year of age. oz = ounce; T = tablespoon.

[a]See Table 7-8 for food specifications. Specifications address topics such as the added ingredients that are allowed in the infant foods.

[b]At 6 months, introduce these foods one at a time, starting with meat or infant cereal, followed by vegetables, fruits, and bread or crackers in amounts and types that are developmentally appropriate.

[c]As prescribed.

[d]As prepared.

[e]No fruit juice for infants under 12 months of age.

groups, the patterns were designed by (1) basing the amounts of foods in each of the five meal components on guidance provided by MyPyramid (USDA, 2009), (2) specifying a wide variety of vegetables, (3) requiring at least half of the grain foods to be in the form of whole grain-rich products, and (4) controlling calories. The patterns are similar to those recommended by the Institute of Medicine for the National School Lunch Program and the School Breakfast Program (IOM, 2010). Patterns for meals and snacks are addressed separately below.

Patterns for Meals

The meal patterns below are expressed as both weekly and daily patterns. Weekly patterns are especially useful for specifying the variety of vegetables to be offered at lunch and the amounts of grains and lean meats or meat alternates to be offered at breakfast. Daily patterns make it clear what amounts of each food group are consistent from day to day. As stated in Chapter 9, USDA will need to arrange for the development and testing of methods for presenting the meal patterns in easy-to-use formats for providers. Regardless of the manner in which they are expressed, they must incorporate the essential elements that are presented under Meal Requirement Recommendation #2.

Weekly patterns Table 7-2 shows the recommended 5-day weekly patterns for breakfast and lunch/supper by age group. Attention to the footnotes is

TABLE 7-2 Recommended Patterns for Breakfast and Lunch/Supper Covering a 5-Day Week: Amounts[a] of Food by Meal, Age Group, Food Group, and Vegetable Subgroup

	Breakfast				
Food Group[b] (Measure)	1 Year	2–4 Years	5–13 Years	14–18 Years	Adults
Fruit (c)[c]	$1\frac{1}{4}^c$	$2\frac{1}{2}^c$	$2\frac{1}{2}^c$	$2\frac{1}{2}^c$	$2\frac{1}{2}^c$
Vegetable (c)	0	0	0	0	0
Dark green	0	0	0	0	0
Orange	0	0	0	0	0
Legumes	0	0	0	0	0
Starchy	0	0	0	0	0
Other	0	0	0	0	0
Grain/bread (oz eq)[d]	$3\frac{1}{2}$	7	$9\frac{1}{2}$	12	12
Lean meat or meat alternate (oz eq)	$1\frac{1}{2}^e$	3^e	3^e	6^e	3^e
Milk (c)	$2\frac{1}{2}$	$2\frac{1}{2}$	$3\frac{3}{4}$	5	$3\frac{3}{4}$

NOTE: c = cup; oz eq = ounce equivalent.

[a]These amounts of food are to be distributed over 5 days of menus. See Table 7-9 and Appendix K for sample menus planned using these patterns.

[b]See Appendix Table H-1 for a listing of foods by MyPyramid food group and subgroup. See Table 7-8 for applicable food specifications to control calories, reduce sodium, and ensure diet quality. Specifications address topics such as the type of milk, forms of fruit, and fat content of meats.

essential for planning meals that meet the Meal Requirements. For example, the table of food specifications (referred to by footnote b) makes it clear that all milk and yogurt for those ages 2 years or older must be low-fat or nonfat.

Although healthy fats (e.g., vegetable oil, olive oil, soft margarine, mayonnaise, many salad dressings) are not listed as part of the meal patterns, moderate amounts are to be included daily. Healthy fats provide essential fatty acids and vitamin E, and they improve the palatability of meals and aid satiety. The table of food specifications (Table 7-8) lists healthy fats.

Daily patterns Table 7-3 shows the recommended daily amounts of food to be offered at breakfast and lunch/supper, by age group. Footnotes e and f are especially important because they link the daily meal pattern to the weekly pattern.

Patterns for Snacks

Regular snacks Regular snacks are small snacks. Most programs provide two meals and one regular snack under CACFP, but programs currently have the option of being reimbursed for one meal and two regular snacks. Each of the recommended regular snacks would provide approximately

		Lunch/Supper		
1 Year	2–4 Years	5–13 Years	14–18 Years	Adults
1¼	2½	2½	2½	2½
1¼	2½	5	5	5
¼	½	1	1	1
¼	½	½	½	½
⅛	¼	½	½	½
¼	½	1	1	1
⅜	¾	2	2	2
2½	5	10	12½	10
2½	5	10	12½	10
2½	2½	5	5	5

cNon-starchy vegetables may be substituted for fruit at breakfast. Non-starchy vegetables include all vegetables in Appendix Table H-1 except those listed in the starchy vegetable subgroup.

dAt least half of the grain/bread must be whole grain-rich (see specifications in Table 7-8). Other grains must be enriched.

eLean meat or meat alternates are to be served 3 days per week at breakfast for all age groups. On each of the days without meat or meat alternates, serve an additional ½ oz eq of bread/grain for 1-year-old children and an additional 1 oz eq of bread/grain for all other age groups.

TABLE 7-3 Recommended Daily Meal Patterns for Breakfast and Lunch/Supper: Amounts of Food by Age Group, Meal, and Food Group[a]

Food Group[b] (Measure)	1 Year	2–4 Years	5–13 Years	14–18 Years	Adults
			Breakfast		
Fruit or non-starchy vegetables (cup)[c]	¼	½	½	½	½
Grain/bread (oz eq)[d]	½	1	1½	2	2
			AND		
Lean meat or meat alternate (oz eq)[e]	½	1	1	2	1
			OR		
Grain/bread (oz eq)[d]	1	2	2½	3	3
			AND		
Lean meat or meat alternate (oz eq)[e]	0	0	0	0	0
		(Amounts of grain/bread and meat or meat alternate vary across the week. See footnote e.)			
Milk (cup)	½	½	¾	1	¾
			Lunch/Supper		
Fruit (cup)	¼	½	½	½	½
Vegetable (cup)[f]	¼	½	1	1	1
Grain/bread (oz eq)[d]	½	1	2	2 ½	2
Lean meat or meat alternate (oz eq)[e]	½	1	2	2 ½	2
Milk (cup)	½	½	1	1	1

NOTE: oz eq = ounce equivalent; svgs = servings; wk = week.

[a]See Table 7-9 and Appendix K for sample menus planned using these patterns.

[b]See Appendix Table H-1 for a listing of foods by food group and subgroup. See Table 7-8 for applicable food specifications to control calories, reduce sodium, and ensure diet quality. Specifications address topics such as the type of milk, forms of fruit, and fat content of meats.

[c]Non-starchy vegetables include all vegetables in Appendix Table H-1 except those listed in the starchy vegetable subgroup.

[d]At least half of the grain/bread must be whole grain-rich. Other grain/bread must be enriched.

[e]Meat/meat alternates should be served 3 days per week at breakfast for all age groups. On each of the days without meat or meat alternates, serve an additional ½ oz eq of bread/grain for children age 1 year and an additional 1 oz eq of bread/grain for all other age groups.

[f]The number of cups indicated represents the total amount of vegetables served at lunch/supper. Offer two different vegetables per meal. With reference to either lunch or supper (or both), serve dark green vegetables at least twice per week, orange vegetables at least twice per week, legumes at least once per week, starchy vegetables no more than twice per week, and other vegetables at least three times per week. *See Appendix Table H-1 for listings of vegetables in each subgroup.* (emphasis added)

one-half as many calories as the lunch meal. Table 7-4 shows the weekly pattern for the regular snack, by age group.

The following three steps provide guidance for using the regular snack pattern:

TABLE 7-4 Weekly Meal Pattern for Regular Snacks: Number of Servings from Each Food Group per Week and Amount per Serving, by Age Group[a]

Food Group[b]	1 Year	2–4 Years	5–13 Years	14–18 Years	Adults
	Number of Servings per Week (Amount/Serving)[c]				
Fruit	2 (½ c)	2 (½ c)	2 (½ c)	2 (1 c)	2 (1 c)
Orange vegetable[d]	1 (⅛ c)	1 (¼ c)	1 (½ c)	1 (½ c)	1 (½ c)
Non-starchy vegetable[e]	1 (⅛ c)	1 (¼ c)	1 (½ c)	1 (1 c)	1 (½ c)
Grain/bread[f]	2 (½ oz eq)	2 (1 oz eq)	2 (1 oz eq)	2 (2 oz eq)	2 (1 oz eq)
Lean meat or meat alternate	2 (½ oz eq)	2 (1 oz eq)	2 (1 oz eq)	2 (1 oz eq)	2 (1 oz eq)
Milk	2 (½ c)	2 (½ c)	2 (½ c)	2 (½ c)	2 (½ c)

NOTE: c = cup; oz eq = ounce equivalent.

[a]See Table 7-9 and Appendix K for sample regular snack menus that follow these patterns.

[b]See Appendix Table H-1 for a listing of foods by MyPyramid food group and subgroup. See Table 7-8 for applicable food specifications to control calories, reduce sodium, and ensure diet quality. Specifications address topics such as the type of milk, forms of fruit, and fat content of meats.

[c]The patterns for each age group show number of servings and amount per serving for either a morning or afternoon snack. If both morning and afternoon snacks are provided daily, the same pattern is to be used for each. Over the course of a 5-day week, a total of 10 servings would be offered for the morning snack and the same number for the afternoon snack (if both were provided); 2 servings would be offered for each daily snack.

[d]See Appendix Table H-1 for a list of orange vegetables.

[e]Non-starchy vegetables include all vegetables in Appendix Table H-1 except those listed in the starchy vegetable subgroup.

[f]At least half of the grain/bread must be whole grain-rich (see specifications in Table 7-8). Other grains must be enriched.

1. Plan regular snacks for a 5-day week so that they meet the requirements shown in Table 7-4 for the age group being served.

2. For all age groups, each daily snack will include two servings, but the size of the servings will vary.

3. Use a snack template to simplify the process of meeting the daily and weekly snack requirements. A sample template is shown in Table 7-5 for children ages 5–13 years. Templates for children ages 1 and 2–4 years and for adults could show the same pattern of meal components, but some of the serving sizes would differ. Note that this is just one example of a template for the children. The food groups could be distributed in different ways over the week, but it is essential to make sure that each daily regular snack includes two servings of the size specified for the age group in Table 7-4 and that the total amounts for each food group are served over the week.

TABLE 7-5 Regular Snack Menu Sample Template[a]: Children 5–13 Years

Food Group [b,c]	Monday	Tuesday	Wednesday	Thursday	Friday
Fruit or fruit juice[d]	0	½ c juice	½ c fruit	0	0
Vegetable	0	½ c orange veg	0	0	½ c non-starchy veg[e]
Cereals/grains/ breads[f]	1 oz eq refined grain	0	0	1 oz eq whole grain	0
Lean meat or meat alternate	0	0	1 oz eq	0	1 oz eq
Low-fat or nonfat milk	½ c	0	0	½ c	0

NOTES: c = cup; oz eq = ounce equivalent; veg = vegetable.

[a]This is only one possible distribution of how the meal components may be served across the day and week.

[b]Provide water as a beverage.

[c]See Appendix Table H-1 for a listing of foods by MyPyramid food group and subgroup. See Table 7-8 for applicable food specifications to control calories, reduce sodium, and ensure diet quality. Specifications address topics such as the type of milk, forms of fruit, and fat content of meats.

[d]Juice is an option only if it is 100 percent fruit juice and has not been served at another meal or snack because juice is limited to one serving per day. "Fruit" refers to fresh, frozen, canned, or dried choices that meet specifications (see Table 7-8).

[e]Non-starchy vegetables include all vegetables in Appendix Table H-1 except those listed in the starchy vegetable subgroup.

[f]At least half of the grains served across the week should be whole grain-rich (see specifications in Table 7-8). Other grains must be enriched.

Enhanced snack In the recommended snack patterns for children, the committee included an option for participants ages 5 years and older. In reviewing the pattern of snacks commonly served to CACFP participants, it was clear that the afternoon snacks were much more common than morning snacks. Furthermore, compared with the time between lunch and supper, the period between breakfast and lunch is typically shorter. Thus, for children at least 5 years of age and adults, the recommendation is for providers to have the option of providing an enhanced snack that would be available only as an afternoon snack. The amounts of meal components in the enhanced snack, shown in Table 7-6, are twice the amounts in the regular snack.

The committee does not recommend an enhanced snack option for children under 5 years of age because these children typically consume smaller meals and require relatively smaller snacks in both the morning and the afternoon.

TABLE 7-6 Weekly Pattern for Enhanced Snacks, by Age Group: Number of Servings from Each Food Group per Week and Amount per Serving, by Age Group[a]

Food Group[b]	5–13 Years	14–18 Years	Adults
	Number of Servings per Week (Amount/Serving)[c]		
Fruit	4 (½ c)	4 (1 c)	4 (1 c)
Orange vegetable[d]	2 (½ c)	2 (½ c)	2 (½ c)
Non-starchy vegetable[e]	2 (½ c)	2 (1 c)	2 (½ c)
Grain/bread[f]	4 (1 oz eq)	4 (2 oz eq)	4 (1 oz eq)
Lean meat or meat alternate	4 (1 oz eq)	4 (1 oz eq)	4 (1 oz eq)
Low-fat or nonfat milk	4 (½ c)	4 (½ c)	4 (½ c)

NOTE: c = cup; oz eq = ounce equivalent.

[a]See Table 7-9 and Appendix K for sample regular snack menus that follow these patterns.

[b]See Appendix Table H-1 for a listing of foods by MyPyramid food group and subgroup. See Table 7-8 for applicable food specifications to control calories, reduce sodium, and ensure diet quality. Specifications address topics such as the type of milk, forms of fruit, and fat content of meats.

[c]The patterns for each age group show number of servings and amount per serving covering a 5-day week. Over the course of the 5-day week, a total of 20 servings would be offered. Each enhanced snack includes 4 servings. For children ages 14–18 years, some of the serving sizes are large, and it may be desirable to offer two items within the same food group to equal the specified amount. The committee urges consideration of the enhanced snack option for adults.

[d]See Appendix Table H-1 for a list of orange vegetables.

[e]Non-starchy vegetables include all vegetables in Appendix Table H-1 except those listed in the starchy vegetable subgroup.

[f]At least half of the grain/bread must be whole grain-rich (see specifications in Table 7-8). Other grains must be enriched.

The following three steps provide guidance for using the enhanced snack pattern:

1. Plan enhanced snacks for a 5-day week so that they meet the requirements shown in Table 7-6 for the age group being served.

2. For all age groups, each daily snack will include four servings. For children ages 14–18 years, some of the serving sizes are large, and it may be desirable to offer more than one food within the same food group.

3. Use a snack template to simplify the process of meeting the daily and weekly snack requirements. A sample template is shown for children ages 14–18 years in Table 7-7. Note that the template is an example only. The meal components could be distributed in

TABLE 7-7 Enhanced Snack Menu Sample Template[a]: Children Ages 14–18 Years

Food Group[b,c]	Monday	Tuesday	Wednesday	Thursday	Friday
Fruit or fruit juice[d]	1 c fruit	½ c juice and ½ c fruit	1 c fruit	2 small pieces[e] of fruit	0
Vegetable	0	½ c orange veg and ½ c dark green veg	1 c nonstarchy veg[f,g]	½ c orange veg	½ c nonstarchy veg[f,g]
Cereals/grains/ breads[h]	2 oz eq enriched grain	2 oz eq whole grain	0	2 oz eq enriched grain	2 oz eq whole grain
Lean meat or meat alternate	1 oz eq	1 oz eq	1 oz eq	0	1 oz eq
Low-fat or nonfat milk	½ c	0	½ c	½ c	½ c

NOTES: c = cup; oz eq = ounce equivalent; veg = vegetable.

[a]This is only one possible distribution of how the meal components may be served across the day and week.

[b]Provide water as a beverage.

[c]See Appendix Table H-1 for a listing of foods by MyPyramid food group and subgroup. See Table 7-8 for applicable food specifications to control calories, reduce sodium, and ensure diet quality. Specifications address topics such as the type of milk, forms of fruit, and fat content of meats.

[d]Juice is an option only if it is 100 percent fruit juice and has not been served at another meal or snack because juice is limited to one serving per day. "Fruit" refers to fresh, frozen, canned, or dried choices that meet specifications (see Table 7-8).

[e]Equivalent to 1 cup.

[f]Non-starchy vegetables include all vegetables in Appendix Table H-1 except those listed in the starchy vegetable subgroup.

[g]This may be a combination of two or more raw or cooked vegetables.

[h]At least half of the grains served across the week should be whole grain-rich (see specifications in Table 7-8). Other grains must be enriched.

different ways over the week, but it is essential to make sure that each daily enhanced snack includes the correct number of servings and that the amounts shown in Table 7-6 for the age group are served over the week. Table 7-7 provides examples (on Tuesday and Thursday) of how an enhanced snack could include more than one type of fruit.

FOOD SPECIFICATIONS

The proposed food specifications for infant, child, and adult CACFP participants provided in Table 7-8 were developed as part of the recom-

TABLE 7-8 Proposed Specifications for Foods in the Child and Adult Care Food Program

Food Group	Participant Group	Specifications[a]
Breast milk	Infants, 0–11 months	Breast milk provided by mother and stored by provider in accordance with CACFP standards
Infant formula	Infants, 0–11 months	Iron-fortified infant formula
Infant cereal	Infants, 6–11 months	Iron-fortified infant cereal, instant
Baby food fruits and vegetables	Infants, 6–11 months	Commercial baby food fruits and vegetables without added sugars, starches, or salt (i.e., sodium)—Texture may range from strained through diced. The provider may process foods to the proper consistency using fresh, frozen, or canned fruits and vegetables that contain no added sugars, starches, salt, or fats.
Baby food meats	Infants, 6–11 months	Single major ingredient, commercial baby food meat; without added sugars, starches, vegetables, or salt (i.e., sodium). The provider may process meats to the proper consistency using fresh, frozen, or canned meats that contain no added sugars, starches, salt, or fats.
Fruits		
Juice	Ages 1 y or older	100 percent fruit juice with no added sugars, limited to one serving per day
Fruits	Ages 1 y or older	Any variety of unsweetened fresh fruits; frozen unsweetened fruits; canned fruits that are packed in juice or water; dried fruit (if it does not pose a choking hazard) without added sugars, fats, oils, or salt
Vegetables		
Vegetables	Children and adults	Any variety of fresh, canned, or plain frozen vegetables. Variety is to be encouraged through the weekly food pattern and nutrition education. Starchy vegetables (e.g., white potatoes, corn) are limited in the meal pattern. Vegetables may be boiled, steamed, baked, or stir fried in a small amount of vegetable oil. No deep-fried vegetables.
Grains[b]		
Whole grain-rich	Children and adults	A serving of a whole grain-rich food must be at least the portion size of one grain/bread serving as defined in the USDA Food Buying Guide for Child Nutrition Programs (USDA/FNS, 2008) and FNS Instruction 783-1 (Revision 2), the Grains/Breads Requirement for the Food-Based Menu Planning Alternative in the Child Nutrition Programs (USDA/FNS, 2008, pp. 3-15–3-16), and must meet at least one of the following two specifications:

continued

TABLE 7-8 Continued

Food Group	Participant Group	Specifications[a]
		1. The product includes the following FDA-approved whole grain health claim on its packaging: "Diets rich in whole grain foods and other plant foods and low in total fat, saturated fat, and cholesterol may reduce the risk of heart disease and some cancers" (FDA, 2008).
		2. Product ingredient listing lists whole grain first, specifically:
		a. Nonmixed dishes (e.g., breads, cereals): Whole grains must be the primary ingredient by weight.
		b. Mixed dishes (e.g., pizza, corn dogs): Whole grains must be the primary grain ingredient by weight (a whole grain is the first grain ingredient in the list).
		Whole grain ingredients are those specified in the *HealthierUS School Challenge Whole Grain Resource* guide (USDA/FNS, 2009) and include whole wheat flour, rye flour, brown rice, bulgur, hulled and de-hulled barley, quinoa, oatmeal, and popcorn, among others. (Popcorn is not to be served to young children because of its choking hazard.)
		For foods prepared by the CACFP provider, the recipe is used as the basis for a calculation to determine whether the total weight of whole grain ingredients exceeds the total weight of non-whole grain ingredients. Detailed instructions for this method appear in the *HealthierUS School Challenge Whole Grains Resource* guide (USDA/FNS, 2009).
Breakfast cereals		Ready-to-eat cereals and hot cereals (instant-, quick-, and regular-cooking forms), whether whole grain-rich or enriched [must conform to FDA standard of identity], must contain less than or equal to 21.2 g sucrose and other sugars per 100 g dry cereal (less than or equal to 6 g per dry oz of cereal, as specified in *WIC Food Packages* [IOM, 2006]).
Other baked or fried grain products	Children and adults	Baked or fried grain products that are high in solid fats and added sugars are limited to one serving per week across all eating occasions. Examples of grain foods that are high in solid fats and added sugars and that are commonly served in CACFP include pancakes and waffles served with syrup, muffins and quick breads, sweet rolls, croissants, toaster pastries, donuts, flour tortillas, granola/cereal bars, cookies, brownies, cake, and pie.

Food Group	Participant Group	Specifications[a]
Milk and alternatives		
Milk	Infants, 0–11 months	No milk products (e.g., yogurt, cheese) allowed
	Children (age 1 y)	Whole milk only
	Children (age ≥ 2 y) and adults	Nonfat (skim) and low-fat (1%), no higher fat milks
	Children (age ≥ 5 y) and adults	Nonfat flavored milk containing no more than 22 g of sugar per 8 fl oz is allowed only for children age 5 and older in at-risk afterschool programs[c] and for adults.
Yogurt	Children (age ≥ 2 y) and adults	Yogurt must conform to the FDA's Standard of Identity (21 C.F.R. 131.200) and any updates of these regulations; low-fat yogurt, (21 C.F.R. 131.203); nonfat yogurt, (21 C.F.R. 131.206); plain or flavored; fortified with vitamin D to be comparable to milk; ≤ 17 g of total sugars per 100 g yogurt (40 g/8 oz serving). Yogurt may not contain more than 1% milk fat. May be used as an alternative to either milk or meat no more than once per day.
Soy beverages and other milk substitutes	Children and adults	Soy beverage must meet the standards set in the USDA/FNS Interim Rule for the Special Supplemental Nutrition Program for Women, Infants, and Children (WIC): Revisions in the WIC Food Packages and provide a minimum 8 g of protein, 100 IU for vitamin D and 500 IU for vitamin A, and 276 mg calcium per 8 oz (USDA/FNS, 2007). Low-fat or nonfat unflavored soy beverages for children at least 2 years of age and adults. Flavored soy beverage must be nonfat and may contain no more than 22 g of sugar per 8 fl oz. Other milk substitutes must be fortified as stated for soy beverage above. For children, requests for soy beverage and other milk substitutes must be processed consistent with USDA procedures.
Meat[d] and meat alternates		
Red meats and poultry	Children and adults	Fresh or plain frozen lean beef, pork, lamb, venison, chicken, turkey, other poultry: broiled, roasted, braised, stewed, stir fried in mixed dishes with nonstick spray or vegetable oil. Remove skin from poultry before serving. Limit higher fat meats (e.g., hamburger with ≥ 20% fat, fatty pork).
Fish	Children and adults	Fresh, frozen, or canned fish or seafood. No more than 6 oz (or for children, age-appropriate servings) of albacore tuna per week. Avoid serving shark, swordfish, tilefish, or king mackerel. Choose low-sodium water-pack canned fish.

continued

TABLE 7-8 Continued

Food Group	Participant Group	Specifications[a]
Highly processed red meat, poultry, and fish	Children and adults	Limit highly processed meat, poultry, and fish (including highly salted products and breaded fried products) to one time per week across all eating occasions.
Eggs	Children and adults	If fried or scrambled, cook in vegetable oil or soft margarine rather than in solid fat.
Cheese	Children and adults	Natural cheese. Low-fat cheese is encouraged. No processed cheese, cheese food, or cheese spread because of their higher sodium content and lower content of other nutrients.
Tofu	Children and adults	May not contain added fats, oils, or sodium.
Dried peas, beans, lentil	Children and adults	Dried or canned. Limit those prepared with added solid fat and high sodium content, such as pork and beans and most types of refried beans. Choose nonfat versions.
Nuts, peanut butter	Children (age 1–3 y)	Nut butters if they do not pose a choking hazard; no nuts
	Children (age ≥ 3 y) and adults	Nut butters and unsalted nuts of any type; preferably with no added salt or sugars; only if measures are taken to avoid choking hazard
Yogurt	Children and adults	See entry under "Milk and alternatives" above.
Healthy fats and oils		
Oils	Children and adults	Moderate amounts of unsaturated vegetable oils such as canola oil, corn oil, olive oil, peanut oil, safflower, sunflower oil
Soft margarine	Children and adults	Moderate amounts of soft vegetable oil table spreads, labeled as containing zero grams of *trans* fat

NOTES: CACFP = Child and Adult Care Food Program; FDA = Food and Drug Administration; FNS = Food and Nutrition Service; g = grams; IU = International Units; mg = milligrams; mo = months; oz = ounce; USDA = U.S. Department of Agriculture; y = years.

[a]Nutrition labels on all foods must state that the content of *trans* fat is zero. Foods that present a choking hazard (e.g., whole grapes, raisins, hot dogs, raw carrots) are not to be offered to young children unless the form of the food has been changed to make it safe for them to eat. See Altkorn et al. (2008) for further information about foods that pose choking hazards.

[b]The meal patterns for children and adults stipulate that at least half the grains served must meet the whole grain-rich food specifications, and an even higher proportion of whole grain-rich grain products is encouraged. All refined grain foods must be enriched.

[c]"At-risk afterschool programs" refers to programs offered by at-risk afterschool care centers: public or private nonprofit organizations that are participating in CACFP as an institution or as a sponsored facility and that provide nonresidential child care to children after school through an approved afterschool care program located in an eligible area.

[d]Weights specified for meat, poultry, and fish in meal patterns refer to edible portion as served.

mended Meal Requirements. Their purpose is to indicate the types of infant foods and foods from the five meal components that will help achieve nutritional quality. In general, the foods are low in solid fats and added sugars (or the frequency of use of such foods is limited). The foods are low in *trans* fat, the use of high-sodium foods is discouraged or limited, some cooking methods are given, and acceptable ingredients are indicated. The committee anticipates that states will develop materials that provide concrete guidance to providers for meeting the specifications.

For reasons of practicality and to limit unfavorable unintended consequences, it may be beneficial for USDA to phase in selected aspects of the food specifications and to have processes in place to test the effects of specific restrictions and for strengthening some of the specifications. A few possibilities follow:

- With regard to grain foods that are high in added sugars (a type of food that the Minute Menu Systems, LLC [2008] data showed was offered frequently), consider setting the initial limit to be two per week rather than one, but set a final date for achieving the goal of no more than once per week.
- Determine how the restriction on flavored milk for young children affects their intake of milk and other foods.
- As acceptable products that are high in whole grain content become more available and affordable, change the specifications for whole grain-rich foods (or increase their proportion in the meal and snack patterns).
- As acceptable products that are lower in sodium become available, increase the specificity for foods with added sodium.

TRANSLATING MEAL REQUIREMENTS INTO MENUS

The committee's recommended Meal Requirements comprise the meal patterns in Tables 7-1 through 7-4 and Table 7-6 together with the proposed food specifications in Table 7-8. Table 7-3 provides one possible method for showing how a daily meal pattern can accurately reflect the weekly pattern. The committee recognizes that tools will need to be developed and tested to simplify the process of translating the Meal Requirements into menus; and, as an example, it provided guidelines for planning snacks for the week, including sample templates (see "Patterns for Snacks" above). To illustrate the result of basing menus on the Meal Requirements, the committee wrote sample menus for breakfast, lunch/supper, and snacks for each age group by calorie level. Table 7-9 shows a 1-week set of sample menus for children ages 5–13 years, and Appendix K presents 2 weeks of sample menus for all the age groups. Although mixed dishes such as stew or gumbo could

TABLE 7-9 Sample Menu for Children Ages 5–13 Years

Food Group	Monday Menu Item	Amt	Tuesday Menu Item	Amt
	Breakfast			
Fruit/juice	Tangerine	½ c	Peaches	½ c
Cereal/grain/ bread	Toasted oats cereal	⅜ c	Oatmeal	¾ c
Additional grain	English muffin	½	WW toast	1 slice
Meat/meat alternate[a]	LF Canadian bacon	1 oz	—	—
Fluid milk	Milk	6 oz	Milk	6 oz
Other items	—	—	Soft margarine	1 tsp
	Lunch/Supper			
Fruit/juice	Pears	½ c	Honey dew melon	½ c
Vegetable	Mixed vegetables	½ c	Green beans	½ c
Additional vegetable	Sweet potatoes	½ c	Cream corn	½ c
Cereal/grain/ bread	WW bun	1.8 oz	WW elbow pasta	1 c
Meat/meat alternate	Chicken burger	2 oz	Beef and pasta casserole (beef)	2 oz
Fluid milk	Milk	8 oz	Milk	8 oz
Other items	Light mayo & ketchup	1 T each	—	—

NOTE: Amt = amount; c = cup; LF = low-fat; oz = ounce; RF = reduced fat; T = tablespoon; tsp = teaspoon; WW = whole wheat.

[a]The committee encourages use of meat alternates whenever possible as an alternative to processed high-sodium meats. Examples could include scrambled egg, natural peanut butter, low-fat yogurt, or low-fat cheese.

be included in menus, the committee named the food items so that readers could easily see how the menus correspond to the menu pattern.

COMPARISON BETWEEN CURRENT AND RECOMMENDED MEAL REQUIREMENTS

The recommended Meal Requirements continue to contain valuable features of the current meal requirements, such as focusing on food groups, specifying minimum amounts of foods to be provided at meals and snacks, and not allowing foods such as soft drinks and candy to qualify for reimbursement. On the other hand, they differ in many important

Wednesday		Thursday		Friday	
Menu Item	Amt	Menu Item	Amt	Menu Item	Amt
Breakfast					
Strawberries	½ c	Diced pears	½ c	Tropical fruit	½ c
LF flour		Choice of			
tortilla	1.1 oz	dry cereal	1 ⅛ c	WW pancakes	1.7 oz
—	—	WW bagel	⅓	—	—
Egg	½	—	—	LF turkey sausage	1 oz
Milk	6 oz	Milk	6 oz	Milk	6 oz
—	—	RF cream cheese	1 T	Syrup	1 T
Lunch/Supper					
Watermelon	½ c	Pineapple	½ c	Fresh orange slices	½ c
		tidbits			
Pinto beans	½ c	Broccoli	½ c	Carrots	½ c
Cabbage	½ c	Cauliflower	½ c	Spinach salad	1 c
Corn tortilla	1.8 oz	Brown rice	1 c	WW noodles	1 c
Chicken		LF Salisbury			
taco (chicken)	2 oz	steak	2 oz	Tuna patties	2 oz
Milk	8 oz	Milk	8 oz	Milk	8 oz
Salsa	2 T	Soft margarine	2 tsp	FF ranch dressing	1 T

ways from those in the current regulations, as shown in Table 7-10. The revisions bring the recommended Meal Requirements in closer alignment with (1) current dietary guidance, (2) regulations for the new WIC food packages, (3) recommendations for competitive foods offered or sold in schools, and (4) recommendations concerning the Meal Requirements for the National School Lunch Program and the School Breakfast Program.

TABLE 7-10 Comparison of Current and Recommended Meal Requirements

Age Groups	Current Requirements	Recommended Requirements and Specifications
Infants	0–3, 4–7, 8–11 mo	0–5, 6–11 mo
Children	Patterns for 3 age groups spanning 1 to 12 years, older children "may be served larger portions"	Patterns for 4 age groups spanning 1 to 19 years
Eating Occasion		
All	Must meet daily pattern	Must meet daily and weekly pattern to provide more flexibility and better alignment with the *Dietary Guidelines*
Breakfast	3 meal components	4 or 5 meal components
Lunch or supper	4 meal components	5 meal components
Snack	Any 2 of 4 components	Variety specified for the week Choice between 2 small snacks or 1 enhanced snack
Meal Component		
Fruit	Fruits and vegetables are combined as a category	Fruits are a separate category, and servings are increased; juice is not provided for infants and is limited for children; fruits containing added sugars are limited.
Vegetable		Vegetables are a separate category from fruit, and servings are increased; must provide variety including dark green leafy, bright yellow/orange, legumes; sodium content is limited; starchy vegetables are limited.
Grain/bread	Enriched or whole grain, proportions not specified	At least half must be whole grain-rich, additional whole grains are encouraged, grain products high in SoFAS are limited to control calories and saturated fat, high-sodium grains are also limited.
Meat/meat alternate	None at breakfast	Included in weekly breakfast pattern three times a week to provide balance to meal but flexibility through the week; some types are limited to help control calories, solid fat, and sodium.
Milk	Any type of fluid milk	Must be nonfat or low-fat (1% fat) for children over 2 years of age and adults. Flavored milk must be nonfat and is allowed only for at-risk afterschool programs[a] and adults. For children over 2 years of age and adults, nonfat or low-fat yogurt may be used as a substitute for milk or as a meat alternate no more than once per day.

Food Component

Energy	No requirement	Calories are controlled by limiting foods high in SoFAS.
Micronutrients	No standard specified by regulation	Meal patterns are designed to achieve, for protein and most micronutrients, DRI targets consistent with a low prevalence of inadequacy.
Fats	No restriction	Label must state zero *trans* fat (if applicable); food specifications limit highly processed and high-fat meats and foods
Sodium	No restriction	No salt at the table; encouragement to prepare foods with less salt. Food specifications limit some sources of sodium.

NOTES: DRI = Dietary Reference Intake; mo = months; SoFAS = solid fats and added sugars.

[a]"At-risk afterschool programs" refers to programs offered by at-risk afterschool care centers: public or private nonprofit organizations that are participating in the CACFP as an institution or as a sponsored facility and that provide nonresidential child care to children after school through an approved afterschool care program located in an eligible area.

Practical Considerations

The recommendations for revised Meal Requirements were influenced by practical considerations relating to the CACFP setting. For example, portion sizes often needed to be rounded up or down to common fractions of 1 cup; and, except for meat and grain at breakfast, the amount to be offered from each major food group at meals was made the same from day to day. Because the committee considers variety from the five vegetable subgroups to be a key element of the Meal Requirements, however, the types of vegetables to be offered must vary from day to day. The committee recognizes that some participants follow a vegetarian meal pattern, and provisions for meat and milk alternates are thus included.

Guidance for Encouraging Breastfeeding

The committee recommends that CACFP providers encourage and support breastfeeding by providing mothers access to breastfeeding education opportunities (such as printed materials, on-line breastfeeding support programs, or pre-recorded audio/visual materials), encouragement to bring a supply of breast milk to the day care site, assurances that the milk will be handled safely, and the opportunity to come to the site to breastfeed the baby when possible. Providers need appropriate storage space for the milk and training in the safe handling and preparation of breast milk for feedings. (Resources for safe handling of milk include ADA [2004] and CDC [2010].) As an additional measure to support breastfeeding, the recommended meal pattern for infants does not provide juice for participants less than 1 year of age or complementary foods before 6 months of age. The committee encourages USDA to work together with other federal agencies as well as state- and local-level coalitions of WIC lactation consultants, and existing breastfeeding programs to consider ways to provide incentives for breastfeeding for both participants and providers. Options for breastfeeding incentives are provided in Appendix L.

SUMMARY

The recommended Meal Requirements encompass (1) daily and weekly meal patterns for breakfast, lunch and supper, and snacks appropriate for the age groups served by CACFP and (2) food specifications to help ensure the nutritional quality of the meals. Key elements of the Meal Requirements for children ages 1 year and older and for adults address (a) the amount of fruit and the amount and type of vegetables to be served; (b) the proportion of grain that is to be whole grain-rich; (c) fruit versus juice; (d) snack components over the course of the week; and (e) limitations on solid fats, added sugars, *trans* fat, and sodium. As described in Chapter 6, the recommendations were designed to align with the *Dietary Guidelines for Americans* and the DRIs with necessary adjustments to keep them practical and to limit cost increases. Encouragement for breastfeeding is strongly supported by the committee. Realistic options for supporting breastfeeding, however, were determined to be beyond the task of making recommendations for revised Meal Requirements.

REFERENCES

AAP (American Academy of Pediatrics). 2009. *Pediatric Nutrition Handbook*, 6th ed. Elk Grove Village, IL: American Academy of Pediatrics.

ADA (American Dietetic Association). 2004. *Infant Feedings: Guidelines for Preparation of Formula and Breastmilk in Health Care Facilities*, edited by S. T. Robbins and L. T. Beker. Chicago, IL: ADA.

Altkorn, R., X. Chen, S. Milkovich, D. Stool, G. Rider, C. M. Bailey, A. Haas, K. H. Riding, S. M. Pransky, and J. S. Reilly. 2008. Fatal and non-fatal food injuries among children (aged 0–14 years). *International Journal of Pediatric Otorhinolaryngology* 72(7):1041–1046.

CDC (Centers for Disease Control and Prevention). 2010. *Proper Handling and Storage of Human Milk*. http://www.cdc.gov/breastfeeding/recommendations/handling_breastmilk. htm (accessed October 21, 2010).

FDA (Food and Drug Administration). 2008. *XI. Appendix C: Health Claims: Guidance for Industry, A Food Labeling Guide*. http://www.fda.gov/Food/GuidanceComplianceRegulatory Information/GuidanceDocuments/FoodLabelingNutrition/FoodLabelingGuide/ ucm064919.htm (accessed November 2, 2010).

HHS/AoA (U.S. Department of Health and Human Service/Administration on Aging). 2006. *Nutrition Service Providers Guide for Older Adults*. Washington, DC: HHS/AoA. http:// www.health.gov/dietaryguidelines/dga2005/toolkit/default.htm (accessed October 11, 2010).

IOM (Institute of Medicine). 2006. *WIC Food Packages: Time for a Change*. Washington, DC: The National Academies Press.

IOM. 2010. *School Meals: Building Blocks for Healthy Children*. Washington, DC: The National Academies Press.

Krebs, N. F., J. E. Westcott, N. Butler, C. Robinson, M. Bell, and K. M. Hambidge. 2006. Meat as a first complementary food for breastfed infants: Feasibility and impact on zinc intake and status. *Journal of Pediatric Gastroenterology and Nutrition* 42(2):207–214.

Minute Menu Systems, LLC. 2008. *Minute Menu Systems*. http://www.minutemenu.com/web/ index.html (accessed August 27, 2010).

USDA (U.S. Department of Agriculture). 2009. *Inside the Pyramid*. http://www.mypyramid. gov/pyramid/index.html (accessed October 19, 2010).

USDA/FNS (U.S. Department of Agriculture/Food and Nutrition Service). 2007. Special Supplemental Nutrition Program for Women, Infants and Children (WIC): Revisions in the WIC Food Packages. Interim Rule. *Federal Register* 72(234);68966–69032.

USDA/FNS. 2008. *Food Buying Guide for Child Nutrition Programs*. Alexandria, VA: USDA/ FNS. http://teamnutrition.usda.gov/Resources/foodbuyingguide.html (accessed November 2, 2010).

USDA/FNS. 2009. *HealthierUS School Challenge Whole Grains Resource*. http://www.fns. usda.gov/TN/HealthierUS/wholegrainresource.pdf (accessed May 14, 2009).

8

Meal Cost Implications

Meal costs encompass food costs plus non-food costs such as labor, supplies, utilities, and the costs of capital and equipment. This chapter focuses primarily on changes in Child and Adult Care Food Program (CACFP) food costs that are projected to result from implementation of the recommended Meal Requirements. The chapter also addresses ways in which specific elements of the recommendations affect those changes and briefly covers non-food meal costs.

PROJECTED CHANGES IN FOOD COSTS

Ideally, the changes in food cost would be estimated by comparing the cost of all food provided through the program before and after the implementation of the recommended Meal Requirements. One approach to obtaining such information is to compare the cost of foods in representative menus planned using the current Meal Requirements with the cost of foods from menus planned using the recommended Meal Requirements; and weighting would be done to reflect the proportions of meals served (by type of meal) to different age groups. Because of a lack of two types of data: (1) current baseline data on a nationally representative sample of meals served by providers, and (2) the distribution of participants by age and meal patterns—the committee used an alternate approach that provides useful, albeit crude, estimates of changes in food costs. This approach is described briefly below and in more detail in Appendix I.

Overview of Methods of Estimation

Baseline Foods

A data set, herein called *CACFP component serving data*,[1] provided data representative of foods used by CACFP family day care providers. Using the CACFP component serving data, the cost estimation process began by grouping the foods currently used by providers into composite food items called *food clusters* and then into composite food groups (composite meal components). The objective of the development of food clusters and composite food groups was to provide a profile of the food currently served by CACFP providers. The first steps included the identification of the food items most commonly offered by providers and weighting of the food items by their current frequency of use for three different meal types (breakfast, lunch/supper, and snack). The weighted composite food groups were then used as a proxy for menus of foods offered and, hence, as the baseline for the evaluation of changes to the food cost[2] of the meals and snacks served. The identified foods and their weights within the clusters were used in the estimation of the cost of the food clusters. In turn, the relative weights of the clusters that belong in each of the current four meal components, estimated separately by eating occasion, allowed the estimation of the baseline cost of each of the meal components by eating occasion. As an example, the "vegetables and fruit" component (a composite food group) offered for breakfast under the current Meal Requirements includes the following weights of seven food clusters: bananas, 23 percent; strawberries/berries/ kiwi, 11 percent; peaches/apricots, 8 percent; oranges, 7 percent; applesauce, 7 percent; pears, 6 percent; various juices, total of 14 percent; and other vegetables and fruits. Price data were applied to the food items within each cluster to obtain the cost of the food clusters.

Foods Representing the Recommended Meal Requirements

Estimates of costs representing the recommended Meal Requirements need to reflect the revised meal patterns and food specifications presented in Chapter 7. To accomplish this, it was necessary to make adjustments in the baseline food clusters and composite food groups, as described in Appendix I. In general, the revised food clusters contain fewer food items that are high in solid fats, added sugars, and/or sodium. Compared to baseline,

---

[1] See Appendix I for information about this data set.

[2] The composite food groups were also used for nutrient analyses; see Chapter 10.

the composite food groups (meal components) for the recommended Meal Requirements differ substantially in several ways:

- Fruits and vegetables are separate meal components;
- The vegetable food group composite contains higher percentages of green vegetables, orange vegetables, and legumes and lower percentages of starchy and other vegetables;
- The fruit food group contains a smaller share of fruit juice at breakfast and snack;[3]
- The grain group contains a higher percentage of whole grain-rich foods;
- The grains and meat/meat alternate group contain lower percentages of food clusters that are high in solid fats and/or added sugars; and
- The milk group contains predominantly plain low-fat and nonfat milk but also a small proportion of yogurt and, for snacks only, flavored milk.

Changes in Amounts of Foods by Meal and Age Group

To estimate changes in food costs, it was necessary to determine the changes in the required amounts of the meal components. This involved a somewhat complex process because of recommended changes in the age groups, the separation of the current fruit/vegetable meal component into fruits and vegetables as two separate meal components, some lack of specificity in the current amounts of food to be served to children older than 12 years, and provider choice of which two meal components to serve in the snack under the current regulations. Table 8-1 shows how the amounts of the meal components change at specific ages for children ages 1–12 years for lunch/supper. Changes for youth ages 13–18 years are not included specifically because the current program specifies that they should receive the same pattern for children ages 6–12 years but with larger portions. Appendix Table I-3 shows the changes in amounts that apply to adults. The changes in amounts of foods served as snacks relied on the use of data provided to the committee concerning the distribution of the four current meal components among snacks served by family day care providers (see Appendix Table I-2). All comparisons in this chapter are between the current snack and the recommended *regular* snack. See Chapter 7 for a description of the proposed *enhanced* snack that would provide more food

---

[3]Essentially no fruit juice was included in either composite at lunch.

TABLE 8-1 Weekly Changes in Amounts of Meal Components in Lunch/ Supper in Recommended Meal Patterns for Children Ages 1 Through 13[a] Years of Age, Compared with Current CACFP Meal Pattern Amounts

Meal Component	1 Year	2 Years	3–4 Years	5 Years	6–13 Years
	Difference: Recommended Minus Current Amounts				
Fruit and vegetables (c)	1¼	3¾	2½	5	3¾
Grains (oz eq)	0	2½	2½	7½	5
Meat/meat alternate (oz eq)	−2½[b]	0	−2½[b]	2½	0
Milk (c)	0	0	−1¼[b]	1¼	0

NOTE: c = cup; CACFP = Child and Adult Care Food Program; oz eq = ounce equivalent.

[a]A clear comparison is not possible for patterns that apply to youth ages 13–18 years because current requirements specify the use of the pattern for children ages 6–12 years but with larger portions.

[b]Negative values indicate a decrease in amounts compared to current practice.

SOURCE: Data on current CACFP meal patterns from USDA/FNS, 2010.

to participants in the at-risk afterschool program. The process used to calculate the cost changes by meal and age group is described in Appendix I.

Sample Menus

As discussed in Chapter 7, sample menus were written following the recommended Meal Requirements. The costs of the sample menus were estimated using the same source for food prices that had been used for the food items in the revised composites (see Appendix I).

Results

Estimated Food Costs of Meals and Snacks

The food costs of meals and snacks under the current and recommended Meal Requirements, as estimated from the current and revised meal component composites, are shown in Table 8-2 by eating occasion and age group. (Appendix Table I-4 provides information illustrating how these cost estimates were made for children ages 2–4 years—the age group with the largest number of participants receiving meals.) The percentage change in food cost is also shown. Except for infants (breakfast for ages 0–5 months and lunch/supper for all infants), the food cost of the meals is substantially higher under the recommended Meal Requirements. The food cost of the regular snack is higher than the baseline cost for children ages 1–4 years and for youths 14–18 years. For the other groups, the food cost of the regular snack is lower or the same as the baseline cost. Notably, the estimated

TABLE 8-2 Comparison of the Daily Costs of Baseline Meal Patterns with Revised Recommended CACFP Meal Patterns Estimated Using Baseline and Revised Meal Component Composites and 2003–2004 Price

Age Group	Cost of Breakfast ($)			Cost of Lunch/Supper ($)			Cost of Standard Snack ($)		
	Baseline	Recommended[a]	% Difference	Baseline	Recommended[a]	% Difference	Baseline[b]	Recommended[a]	% Difference
Infants 0–5 mo	0.95	0.85	-11	1.05	0.85	-19	0.85	0.85	0
Infants 6–11 mo	1.27	1.30	2	1.43	1.39	-3	0.80	0.57	-29
Children 1 y	0.28	0.45	61	0.46	0.58	26	0.23	0.24	4
Children 2–4 y	0.40	0.66	65	0.65	0.89	37	0.23	0.29	26
Children 5–13 y	0.59[c]	0.73	24	1.07[c]	1.51	41	0.38[c]	0.33	-13
Children 14–18 y	0.70[d]	1.03	47	1.28[d]	1.65	29	0.39[d]	0.51	31
Adults	0.70[e]	0.83	19	1.28[e]	1.56	22	0.39[e]	0.40	3

NOTES: CACFP = Child and Adult Care Food Program; mo = month; y = year(s).

[a]For the method of estimating the costs of the recommended meal patterns by using costs for meal component composites, see Appendix I.

[b]The cost of the baseline standard snack considered the distribution of meal components shown in Table I-2 in Appendix I.

[c]These costs are the average of the costs for the meal component composites for children ages 5–10 and 11–13 years.

[d]Baseline cost relies on assumptions about serving amounts because current regulations specify only that children ages 12 and older may be served larger portions than required for the child meals and snacks based on their greater food needs, but no less.

[e]There were no baseline composite data for adults so the cost of the 14–18-year-olds' menus were used for comparison.

SOURCE: Cost data based on representative food composites from Minute Menu Systems (based on data obtained from family day care homes during August 2009 and February 2010) (Minute Menu Systems, LLC, 2008), and USDA/CNPP Price Database, 2003–2004 prices (USDA/CNPP, 2009) (see Appendix I).

costs of the sample menus were slightly higher for breakfast and snacks and lower for lunch/supper than the cost estimates that were derived using the revised composites (see Appendix Table I-5). Even so, the committee recognizes that the adoption of all the recommended changes in the Meal Requirements would result in a substantial increase in food cost overall.

Amounts of Food as Related to Changes in Food Costs

The changes in the amounts of food required account for a majority of the changes in food costs, as summarized below:

- The lower or near-constant cost for the feedings of infants is the net effect of changes in the amount of iron-fortified infant formula and solid foods for the younger infants.
- The lower cost for the snacks of infants ages 6–11 months results primarily from the reduction in the amount of infant formula.[4]
- The higher cost of meals for children ages 1 year or older and for adults results from changes in the amounts and types of foods to be offered. The major differences are increases in the total amount of fruits and vegetables, especially at lunch; in the amount of grains for some age groups at both breakfast and lunch; and the inclusion of a meat/meat alternate at some breakfasts. The increases are only partially offset by lower amounts of meat/meat alternates for the 1-year-old and 3–4-year-old children at lunch.[5]
- The lower cost of the revised regular snack for infants, children ages 5–13 years, and adults results mainly from the smaller size of the snack (and less formula for infants). Compared with the current snack for all the age groups except children ages 14–18 years, the revised snack provides smaller amounts of food, but the snack pattern specifies more variety. Table I-2 in Appendix I shows that currently the snacks include a grain food, the least expensive food group, as one of the two items nearly half of the time. It is not possible to make a one-to-one comparison of the amounts of food provided by the current snack pattern with either the proposed regular or enhanced snack pattern because providers currently choose which two of the four items to offer. For both the regular and enhanced recommended snack patterns, there is specificity regarding the meal components and food subgroups that are to be used over the week.

---

[4]This is the amount of formula that is allowed for reimbursement. Providers could offer more if needed.

[5]The lower amounts relate to the change in the age groupings.

Changes in Cost by Age Groups

The committee was unable to estimate the average increase in the cost of meals and snacks across all the age groups served because data were lacking on the distribution of the meals and snacks served across the eating occasions by age group. As shown in Chapter 2, Table 2-3, the distribution of participants in different settings is very uneven, with the largest number in child care and the smallest number in adult day care. Very limited evidence suggests that, for young children, the majority of CACFP providers seek reimbursement for two meals and one snack (Personal communication, J. Hirschman, August 2–4, 2010). Data on the distribution of meals and snacks from the 1997 U.S. Department of Agriculture (USDA) Food and Consumer Service (FCS) Early Childhood and Child Care Study (USDA/FCS, 1997) are of limited value, especially because the study preceded the Child Nutrition Reauthorization Act of 1998, which authorized reimbursement for snacks for children up to age 18 in afterschool care programs.

Consequently, the estimates of changes in costs of meal combinations presented here are restricted to those applicable to the two largest groups being served—(1) young children and (2) youth in at-risk afterschool programs—and to specified meal combinations (see Table 8-3).

As expected, the costs of the meal combinations reflect the underlying changes in the individual meal costs. The lower or relatively small increases in the cost of the regular snack are outweighed by increases in the cost of supper. Serving the enhanced snack rather than one regular snack with supper would greatly increase the cost to providers for the at-risk afterschool care program. The estimated cost of the enhanced snack is twice that of the regular snack, namely $0.66 for 5–13-year-olds, $1.02 for 14–18-year-olds, and $0.80 for adults. This means, for example, there would be an

TABLE 8-3 Estimated Cost Changes for CACFP Meals and Snacks Served to Children Ages 1–4 Years and to Youth Ages 5–18 Years Given Specified Meal Combinations

Age Group	Meal Combinations	Change in Cost ($)	Percentage Change in Cost (%)
1 y	Breakfast, lunch, and snack	0.30	31
2–4 y	Breakfast, lunch, and snack	0.56	44
5–13 y	Regular snack and supper	0.39	27
14–18 y	Regular snack and supper	0.49	29

NOTE: CACFP = Child and Adult Care Food Program; y = year(s).
SOURCE: Cost data based on representative food composites from Minute Menu Systems, LLC (based on data obtained from family day care homes during August 2009 and February 2010) (Minute Menu Systems, LLC, 2008) and USDA/CNPP Price Database, 2003–2004 prices (USDA/CNPP, 2009) (see Appendix I).

additional $0.51 cost to serve an enhanced snack instead of a regular snack to the 14–18-year-olds.

Factors Contributing to the Increased Food Cost

In view of the substantial increase in food cost that would be expected to result from recommendations that improve the alignment of CACFP meals with the *Dietary Guidelines*, the committee performed three additional analyses. The intent was to provide information that could be useful to USDA in determining cost-cutting measures, if necessary. The first analysis provides estimates for the change in costs of the baseline and revised meal component composites, by eating occasion (Table 8-4), using data for the largest age group (2–4 years). The second analysis provides estimates of the range of unit costs of the revised meal components by eating occasion, across all the age groups except infants (Table 8-5). The third analysis provides estimates of the cost per standard unit for selected meal component subgroups and of selected grain foods that would be increased or decreased in the recommended meal patterns (Table 8-6).

Change in Unit Cost of the Composites

The unit costs of the baseline breakfast, lunch, and snack composite differ because different foods were included in the composites at the different

TABLE 8-4 Comparison of Average Unit Cost ($) of Baseline Meal Component Composites and Composites Revised to Align with Recommended Meal Requirements[a] for Children Ages 2–4 Years, Based on 2003–2004 Prices

Meal Component	Unit	Breakfast Composites		Lunch/Supper Composites		Snack Composites	
		Baseline	Revised	Baseline	Revised	Baseline	Revised
Fruits and vegetables	1 c[b]	0.44	00.47	0.55	0.77	0.23	0.39
Grain	1 oz eq	0.12	0.17	0.08	0.09	0.14	0.14
Meat/meat alternate	1 oz eq	NA[c]	0.22	0.17	0.18	0.20	0.19
Milk	8 fl oz	0.23	0.24	0.22	0.19	0.22	0.23

NOTE: c = cup; fl oz = fluid ounce; oz eq = ounce equivalent.

[a]For the method of estimating the cost of the menu component composites, see Appendix I.

[b]This value represents the amount of fruits and vegetables combined.

[c]The current breakfast pattern does not include meat/meat alternate.

SOURCE: Cost data based on representative food composites from Minute Menu Systems, LLC (based on data obtained from family day care homes during August 2009 and February 2010) (Minute Menu Systems, LLC, 2008) and USDA/CNPP Price Database, 2003–2004 prices (USDA/CNPP, 2009) (see Appendix I).

TABLE 8-5 Range[a] of Mean Cost (\$) for One Serving of Each of the Five Revised Meal Components, by Eating Occasion

Meal Component	Range of Serving Sizes	Breakfast	Lunch/Supper	Snack
Fruit	¼–½ c	0.12–0.23	0.13–0.26	0.20–0.40
Vegetables	⅛–½ c	NA[b]	0.07–0.26	0.04–0.16
Grain	½–2½ oz eq	0.06–0.24	0.05–0.23	0.07–0.27
Meat	½–2½ oz eq	0.11–0.45	0.09–0.46	0.10–0.19
Milk	½–1 c	0.12–0.24	0.09–0.19	0.11–0.18

NOTE: c = cup; NA = not applicable; oz eq = ounce equivalent.

[a]The range covers the range of serving sizes for the age groups, excluding infants, and may vary by eating occasion.

[b]The revised meal pattern allows for either fruit or non-starchy vegetables at breakfast, but the revised breakfast composite includes only fruit.

SOURCE: Cost data based on representative food composites from Minute Menu Systems, LLC (based on data obtained from family day care homes during August 2009 and February 2010) (Minute Menu Systems, LLC, 2008) and USDA/CNPP Price Database, 2003–2004 prices (USDA/CNPP, 2009) (see Appendix I).

TABLE 8-6 Unit Costs[a] for Selected Types of Foods That Are Recommended in Increased or Decreased Amounts

Food Component	Food Increased in Amount	Unit	Unit Cost (\$)[a]	Food Decreased in Amount	Unit	Unit Cost (\$)
Fruit	Fruit (fresh, canned, dried)	1 c	0.49	Fruit juice	1 c	0.22
Vegetables	Dark green vegetables	1 c	0.78	Starchy vegetables	1 c	0.72
	Orange vegetables	1 c	0.33	Other vegetables	1 c	0.40
	Legumes	1 c	0.25			
Grains	Whole grain bread	1 oz eq	0.10	Refined bread and crackers	1 oz eq	0.09
	Whole grain cereal	1 oz eq	0.16	Refined grain cereal	1 oz eq	0.09
Meat/meat alternate	Chicken cluster with baked chicken[b]	1 oz eq	0.18	Chicken cluster with frozen chicken nuggets[b]	1 oz eq	0.16

NOTE: c = cup; oz eq = ounce equivalent.

[a]Unit costs for food subgroup composites, except fruit juices, whole grain cereal and refined grain cereal, are based on the revised composites for the lunch/supper meal and 2003–2004 prices. Unit costs for fruit juice, whole grain cereal, and refined grain cereal are based on the revised composites for the breakfast meal and 2003–2004 prices.

[b]As an example of the changes in the meat/meat alternate group, the chicken food composite was modified from the original to reduce the share of frozen chicken nuggets in the chicken composite. This change increased the unit cost from \$0.16 to \$0.18.

SOURCE: Cost data based on representative food composites from Minute Menu Systems, LLC (based on data obtained from family day care homes during August 2009 and February 2010) (Minute Menu Systems, LLC, 2008) and USDA/CNPP Price Database, 2003–2004 prices (USDA/CNPP, 2009) (see Appendix I).

eating occasions. The same is true for the costs of the revised composites. As shown in Table 8-4, when the costs of the revised composites were compared with those of the representative baseline composites, either no changes or relatively small changes were found. The biggest increases in unit costs of the revised meal components occurred as a result of recommended changes in the foods included in the fruit/vegetables (at breakfast, lunch/supper, and snack) and the grain groups (excluding snacks). In the revised breakfast and snack composites, a substantial (> 50 percent) reduction in the proportion of fruit that is juice[6] influenced the degree of the difference. The substantial increase in the unit cost of the revised fruit and vegetable composites is largely due to the increased variety of vegetables. The increase in unit costs of the fruit and vegetable and grain components means that the recommended forms of the foods in these components (e.g., the variety of vegetables and the increase in whole grain-rich foods) contribute to the increased cost: the *amounts* of these meal components account for most, but not all, of the increase in food cost by eating occasion and age group. The increased variety of vegetables at lunch/supper contributes to the cost of the revised composite, with an increase of more than 20 percent. Because only the most commonly consumed fruits and vegetables and currently used whole grains were included in the baseline and revised components (in different proportions), it is possible that expanding the variety of fruits and vegetables served or including new and different whole grains would change the estimated cost of the revised composite.

Range of Costs of the Meal Components

Table 8-5 shows the range of serving sizes and costs of specific meal components for each of the three eating occasions. The average cost of one-fourth cup of fruit at breakfast, for example, was $0.12, but the average cost of the same amount (but a different selection) of fruit at snack was $0.20. By looking at this table, one can see that increasing the amount of vegetables by one-half cup at lunch/supper contributes approximately $0.26 extra to the cost of the meal.

Unit Costs for Selected Types of Food

Table 8-6 shows how average unit costs differ for selected types of foods. For example, on average, a 4-ounce portion of fruit is more expensive than 4 ounces of juice; dark green vegetables are more expensive than the other types of vegetables; and whole grain products are slightly more expensive than refined grain products. The table makes it clear that specifying limits on the proportion of fruit that may be in the form of fruit juice,

---

[6]Juice is the less expensive form of fruit; see Table 8-5.

increasing the proportion of specific types of vegetables, and specifying that at least half the grain must be whole grain-rich all contribute to increased food costs. In addition, changes in some of the composites to limit saturated fat also contribute to increased food costs. For example, Table 8-6 shows the effects of substituting a baked chicken cluster for chicken nuggets.

"What-If?" Scenarios

Using the information above, one can obtain a rough estimate of what effect various changes would have on the cost of a recommended meal for a specified age group. For example:

- If the amount of fruit per week at lunch were reduced by half for the 2–4-year age group (from 2.5 to 1.25 cups per week, which is equivalent to a decrease from 0.5 to 0.25 cups per day), then the cost would be reduced by about $0.65 per week. This estimate uses the lunch/supper price for fruit ($0.26 for 0.5 cup, from Table 8-5). $0.26 × 5 days = $1.30 per week, half of which would be $0.65.

- If 0.5 cup of juice were served in place of fruit at a meal or snack, then the cost would be reduced by about $0.68 per week ([$0.49–$0.22 = $0.27 per cup from Table 8-6] × 5 days = $1.35 per cup, or $0.68 per half cup, half of which would be $0.68, from Table 8-6).

- If a whole grain-rich food were substituted for the meat at breakfast for the 2–4-year age group, then the cost would be reduced by half for those ages 5 years and older, about $0.24 per week. (The pattern calls for 1 ounce of meat at breakfast three times per week for this age group. Taking the composite cost of meat from Table 8-5 [$0.22] and the average of whole grain bread and cereal from Table 8-6 [$0.14 with rounding], one subtracts the cost of the grain from the cost of the meat and multiplies the result times 3 days: [$0.22–$0.14] × 3 days.)

- If the vegetables at lunch were reduced by half for those ages 5 years and older (to 0.5 cups per day total) and the same variety were maintained, then the cost would be reduced by $0.26 per day or $1.30 per week.

In all these examples, the decrease in cost is accompanied by movement away from alignment with *Dietary Guidelines* and lower intake of nutrients and/or fiber.

Summary of Effects of Recommended Meal Requirements on Food Cost

Overall, the major changes that lead to the substantial increase in food cost are

1. Increased amount and variety of vegetables at lunch;
2. Increased use of whole fruit and decreased use of juice, especially for the snacks;
3. Larger percentage of whole grain-rich grain products at all eating occasions; and
4. Addition of lean meat or meat alternate to the breakfast meal.

By contrast, changes that slightly offset the cost increases are

1. Smaller amounts of infant formula for infants, at all meals (and snacks for the older infants), and elimination of solid foods for the younger infants;
2. Some reduction of the meat or meat alternate for younger children at lunch; and
3. Reduction in the amount of food offered in standard snacks for children above the age of 5 years.

When developing the meal patterns, the committee considered the effect on costs of increasing the amounts and types of foods to be recommended but gave priority to improving alignment with *Dietary Guidelines*.

Limitations of the Analyses

The committee recognizes a number of limitations to the cost analyses that result from the lack of appropriate baseline data both for determining baseline meals served and for distributing aggregate costs across the different age groups:

- No recent nationally representative data exist on foods served in CACFP meals. The current meal requirements offer providers relatively large scope and flexibility in the selection of foods within the required components. In addition, providers select their own methods of food preparation and use of condiments, and they may serve other (unreimbursed) foods.
- The food composite database for food costs covers only foods served by family day care homes, which provide care for children. These homes constitute 73 percent of CACFP facilities. The committee assumed that the foods selected by the homes are foods that are "economical" for the providers and selected to meet the existing program criteria. The prices used in determining the cost of foods were prices associated with foods consumed in households and prepared at home. However, to the extent that child care centers, afterschool programs, and adult day care currently serve foods

that differ from those used in a "home" setting or face different prices for food because of their ability to access different markets or purchase in larger quantities, the estimates for the changes in cost will differ. For example, the larger child care centers may have access to some savings through bulk (case) purchase of food items, and this may affect the type of food selected and the cost. Moreover, in a limited number of states, some centers (but not family day care homes) may have access to USDA foods (previously called commodity foods), including fruits, vegetables, and whole grain-rich products. The use of these foods would reduce the estimated increase in food costs (IOM, 2010).

- Numerous assumptions were required when determining the food clusters for the baseline meal patterns and modifying these clusters for the recommended meal patterns. To the extent possible when making the revisions, only necessary and limited modifications were made to the baseline food clusters under the assumption that these foods served were well accepted by participants. Implementation of the recommended Meal Requirements may lead to additional changes in the selection of foods offered.

- Price changes for different foods have not been uniform over the years since 2003–2004 (IOM, 2010; Monsivais et al., 2010). Differential price changes may have increased or decreased the effect of the recommended changes in food groups on the net change in cost and, hence, on the cost of foods served by providers.

- The overall effect on the change of food cost for the program (considering all age groups) needs to take account of the relative number of participants for each meal type by age group. The lack of data on the distribution of types of meals limited the ability of the committee to estimate the aggregate food costs associated with offering meals.

NON-FOOD MEAL COSTS

The following discussion of non-food meal costs that are covered by the federal meal reimbursements does not include administrative costs, which averaged about 6 percent of total program cost from fiscal year (FY) 2005 through FY 2009 (Personal communication, E. Harper, July 30, 2010).

The cost of food represents only a portion of the providers' costs for meals and snacks. No studies were found that document the average proportions of total costs to attribute to food, labor, and other costs among providers who participate in CACFP. Data from the second School Lunch and Breakfast Cost Study (USDA/FNS, 2008) indicate that reported costs for operating the school meals programs average about 46 percent for food costs, 45 percent for labor costs, and 10 percent for other costs.[7] These values appear to have limited applicability to CACFP, however, because of substantial differences in the food service operations. According to the Alabama Department of Education Child Nutrition Program (2010), food costs (which include sales taxes and delivery fees) must account for *at least* 50 percent of operating costs.

The costs for menu planning, food acquisition, food preparation, training, and reporting vary widely by provider type. Sponsoring organizations may handle menu planning, training, and much of the record keeping for sponsored centers and for family and group homes; sponsoring organizations for affiliated centers receive separate reimbursement for these services; independent centers do not.

Providers serving small numbers of clients are unlikely to be able to arrange for food delivery and thus incur costs related to the time and transportation needed to shop for the food. These costs could be considerable for small day care sites located in food deserts, because fewer processed foods (a variety of fruits and vegetables, for example) could be obtained only from distant stores, and transportation may be limited (Bodor et al., 2010; IOM, 2009; Rose and Richards, 2004; Sharkey, 2009; Smith and Morton, 2009; Zenk et al., 2009). Note that even uncompensated time, as may occur in family day care homes, has a value.

Although there is no clear basis on which to produce an estimate of the impact of the recommended Meal Requirements on non-food meal costs, the non-food costs are expected to increase at least initially because change will be required. The magnitude and persistence of the increase will vary widely—across the United States, within states, by provider type, and by the quality and amount of technical assistance provided (see Chapter 9). The committee found no data on which to base an estimate of the extent to which increases in non-food meal costs are likely to persist. A single publication (Gabor et al., 2010) addresses increased non-food meal costs in child care. Gabor and colleagues (2010) note that, in Delaware, more food is prepared from basic ingredients to comply with the state's new meal guidelines. As documented by Wagner and colleagues (2007) for the school meal setting, the introduction of more on-site food preparation requires greater managerial skill, may require a one-time investment in equipment, and may require more skilled labor and/or training, but food costs decrease.

Because the recommended Meal Requirements are considerably more detailed than the current ones and because there is substantial turnover among CACFP providers, an increase in training needs (and therefore costs)

---

[7]For many school meal programs, full costs are higher than reported costs because the school district underwrites some costs (USDA/FNS, 2008).

is likely to persist. The training would be supportive of providers' ability to serve appetizing, nutritious meals; provide sound nutrition education to participants and families; and help providers manage their food service safely and efficiently.

SUMMARY

The recommended Meal Requirements increase overall food costs in CACFP mainly because of increased amounts and variety of fruits and vegetables for many age groups at lunch/supper and snacks, the addition of meat/meat alternates at breakfast (balanced only in part by reductions of meat/meat alternates at lunch for the younger children), and increases in the amount of whole grain-rich foods for some age groups. Non-food meal costs are expected to increase initially, to vary with the provider setting and with the extent to which the provider has already implemented changes similar to those recommended, and to be influenced substantially by the quality and extent of technical assistance provided. An increased need for training may persist but will be accompanied by improvements in food service and nutrition education, especially in larger centers.

REFERENCES

Alabama Department of Education Child Nutrition Program. 2010. *Financial Records for CACFP.* http://cnp.alsde.edu/cacfp/CACFPPresentations/10POFinancialRecords.ppt (accessed August 23, 2010).

Bodor, J. N., J. C. Rice, T. A. Farley, C. M. Swalm, and D. Rose. 2010. Disparities in food access: Does aggregate availability of key foods from other stores offset the relative lack of supermarkets in African American neighborhoods? *Preventive Medicine* 51(1):63–67.

Gabor, V., K. Mantinan, K. Rudolph, R. Morgan, and M. Longjohn. 2010. *Challenges and Opportunities Related to Implementation of Child Care Nutrition and Physical Activity Policies in Delaware: Findings from Focus Groups with Child Care Providers and Parents.* Washington, DC: Altarum Institute. http://www.altarum.org/files/pub_resources/DelawareFocusGroup-FullReport-FIN.pdf (accessed July 13, 2010).

IOM (Institute of Medicine). 2009. *The Public Health Effects of Food Deserts.* Washington, DC: The National Academies Press.

IOM. 2010. *School Meals: Building Blocks for Healthy Children.* Washington, DC: The National Academies Press.

Minute Menu Systems, LLC. 2008. *Minute Menu Systems.* http://www.minutemenu.com/web/index.html (accessed August 27, 2010).

Monsivais, P., J. McLain, and A. Drewnowski. 2010. The rising disparity in the price of healthful foods: 2004–2008. *Food Policy* 35(6):514–520.

Rose, D., and R. Richards. 2004. Food store access and household fruit and vegetable use among participants in the US Food Stamp Program. *Public Health Nutrition* 7(8):1081–1088.

Sharkey, J. 2009. Rural food deserts: Perspectives from rural Texas. Presented at the Institute of Medicine-National Research Council Workshop on the Public Health Effects of Food Deserts, Washington, DC, January 26–27.

Smith, C., and L. W. Morton. 2009. Rural food deserts: Low-income perspectives on food access in Minnesota and Iowa. *Journal of Nutrition Education and Behavior* 41(3):176–187.

USDA/CNPP (U.S. Department of Agriculture/Center for Nutrition Policy and Promotion). 2009. *USDA Food Plans: Cost of Food*. http://www.cnpp.usda.gov/usdafoodplanscostof food.htm (accessed August 30, 2010).

USDA/FCS (U.S. Department of Agriculture/Food and Consumer Service). 1997. *Early Childhood and Child Care Study: Nutritional Assessment of the CACFP: Final Report, Volume 2*. Alexandria, VA: USDA/FCS. http://www.fns.usda.gov/ora/menu/Published/CNP/cnp-archive.htm (accessed July 9, 2010).

USDA/FNS (U.S. Department of Agriculture/Food and Nutrition Service). 2008. *School Lunch and Breakfast Cost Study II, Final Report*. Alexandria, VA: USDA/FNS. http://www.fns.usda.gov/OANE/MENU/Published/CNP/FILES/MealCostStudy.pdf (accessed August 4, 2008).

USDA/FNS. 2010. *Child & Adult Care Food Program Meal Patterns*. http://www.fns.usda.gov/cnd/care/ProgramBasics/Meals/Meal_Patterns.htm (accessed March 24, 2010).

Wagner, B., B. Senauer, and F. C. Runge. 2007. An empirical analysis of and policy recommendations to improve the nutritional quality of school meals. *Review of Agricultural Economics* 29(4):672–688.

Zenk, S. N., L. L. Lachance, A. J. Schulz, G. Mentz, S. Kannan, and W. Ridella. 2009. Health promoting community design/nutrition: Neighborhood retail food environment and fruit and vegetable intake in a multiethnic urban population. *American Journal of Health Promotion* 23(4):255–264.

9

Implementation

The effectiveness of the recommended Meal Requirements for the Child and Adult Care Food Program (CACFP) will be determined in large part by two major factors: (1) the manner in which the new requirements are implemented and monitored for compliance and (2) the extent to which the children and adults who are enrolled for care in participating child or adult care facilities consume appropriate amounts of the foods that are offered. Clients' consumption of the food served (the second factor) will be strongly influenced by the implementation methods that are used (the first factor). The first section of this chapter focuses on ways to promote the implementation of key elements of the recommended Meal Requirements. The second section addresses technical assistance pertaining to engaging stakeholders, menu planning, controlling costs, and meeting reporting requirements. The third section addresses the need for revisions to reporting requirements and monitoring procedures. The fourth section presents specific recommendations to support the implementation of the recommended Meal Requirements. The fifth section considers options for updating the Meal Requirements in response to future changes in the *Dietary Guidelines for Americans* (HHS/USDA, 2005) and the Dietary Reference Intakes (DRIs).

Food service operations vary widely across CACFP settings. As used in this chapter, the term *food service operation* refers to preparation facilities that range from home kitchens in day care homes, to small "mom and pop"-type facilities, to large institutional kitchens. In a large majority of the CACFP settings, the facilities, personnel, and other resources are much more limited than those in school meals programs.

PROMOTING THE IMPLEMENTATION OF KEY ELEMENTS
OF THE RECOMMENDED MEAL REQUIREMENTS

Overview

Implementation of the key elements of the recommended Meal Requirements for CACFP (see section "Recommended Meal Requirements" in Chapter 7) will require many changes on the part of providers, sponsoring organizations, state agencies, and organizations that develop educational materials and offer training for CACFP providers. The committee recognizes that changes in Meal Requirements to meet *Dietary Guidelines* increase the complexity and cost of being a CACFP provider and introduce foods that may be unfamiliar to many clients. Two major concerns are that implementation of the new Meal Requirements may negatively affect participation by (1) care providers and (2) clients. Especially in the current economy, any loss of revenue based on decreased participation by clients or increased costs to providers would present a real threat to the financial stability of the program. Providers may themselves be economically challenged while serving mainly low-income younger children or low-income disabled and older adults. Reduced participation in CACFP by care providers would weaken the food safety net and could have negative effects on the nutrition of those needing care.

Therefore, careful consideration needs to be given to the many aspects of implementing change. A plan that introduces change incrementally over a realistic time frame—one developed with the involvement of key stakeholders—may be an important step in the successful implementation of the new Meal Requirements.

Measures to Increase the Feasibility of Implementing Key Elements of the Meal Requirements

This section covers (1) implementing key elements for infants, (2) measures to address key elements for those ages 1 year and older, and (3) measures that are more general in scope. A sample of the many resources that may be tapped to assist with implementation efforts is presented in Appendix M.

Implementing Key Elements for Infants

For infants, the key elements of the new Meal Requirements involve delaying the introduction of infant meats, cereals, vegetables, and fruits until the age of 6 months and the omission of fruit juice of any type before 1 year of age. These changes are expected to be feasible right away, in large part because they bring CACFP into alignment with the food packages and education provided by the Supplemental Nutrition Program for Women, Infants, and Children.

Implementing Key Elements for Clients Ages 1 Year and Older

This subsection first addresses general factors that may foster clients' acceptance of the recommended changes in foods offered. Second, it covers measures to address the availability of suitable foods in food deserts (neighborhoods and communities that have limited access to affordable and nutritious foods [IOM, 2009]). Then, it covers each of the key elements individually. Cost is addressed separately in the section "Controlling Costs." The committee recognizes that a large proportion of providers may already have incorporated many of these measures into their care settings but anticipates that many providers may need to adopt new or improved approaches to successfully implement the key elements of the recommended Meal Requirements.

Fostering clients' acceptance of change In general, food consumption is fostered by the appropriate timing of meals, adequate time for eating the meal, suitable style of meal service, positive interactions with adults during mealtime for younger children, pleasant eating spaces, the availability of assistance with eating and texture modifications for those with chewing or swallowing difficulties, and the scheduling of playtime for younger children or free unstructured relaxed time for the adults. To the extent that foods new to providers are to be incorporated into menus, the providers will need to become familiar with easy, tasty, and appealing ways to prepare and serve them. In addition, menu items need to be developmentally, geographically, and culturally appropriate. For children, repeated exposures to new foods over time improve their preference for those foods (Birch, 1987; Birch and Marlin, 1982). Although waste will occur when children are introduced to foods, it is developmentally appropriate to continue to offer the food. Involving child and adult participants, families or other regular care givers, and CACFP staff members in taste-testing new food items or recipes may be helpful.

Increasing the amount and variety of vegetables To provide the most practical approach to ensuring a suitable variety of vegetables over the week, strategies will need to be developed and tested. To foster acceptance of a variety of vegetables, steps can be taken to make them more appealing in appearance, taste, and texture. A number of studies have documented that repeated exposure to fruit and vegetables results in higher preference for and/or intake of those foods (Bere and Klepp, 2005; Brug et al., 2008; Cooke, 2007; Cullen et al., 2003; Neumark-Sztainer et al., 2003; Wardle et al., 2003). The U.S. Department of Agriculture (USDA) could explore how the lessons learned from initiatives such as the Fresh Fruit and Vegetable Program can inform the implementation of this key element. The committee is aware of anecdotal reports of the positive impact of the exposure to fresh fruits and vegetables on children, families, and the local community (e.g., expansion into grocery stores).

Increasing the proportion of whole grain-rich foods Based on studies that have demonstrated that an incremental increase in whole wheat content of food items resulted in favorable whole grain consumption by children (Burgess-Champoux et al., 2006; Chan et al., 2008; Marquart, 2009; Rosen et al., 2008), it is reasonable to expect the acceptance of whole grain-rich foods—especially if they are introduced gradually. Additionally, products made with white whole wheat and other lighter-colored whole grains can be used in place of refined grains, as these types of flour minimize changes in product appearance and thus increase acceptance (Marquart, 2009).

Specifying fruit in place of most juice Many fruit options are available because the fruit may be unsweetened fresh, frozen, canned, or (in some cases) dried. The higher cost of fruit compared with juice may be the major deterrent.

Serving foods that are low in solid fats, *trans* fat, added sugars, and sodium Easy-to-use materials can be developed based on the proposed table of food specifications (Table 7-8 in Chapter 7). The two biggest challenges are expected to be the availability, in any market, of reasonably priced and palatable prepared or partially prepared foods that are low in sodium (IOM, 2010) and a suitable selection of these foods in rural or urban food deserts.

Serving acceptable lean meat or meat alternatives at breakfast A number of suitable choices are available. Examples include low-fat or fat-free yogurt, low-fat cheese, nuts or seeds (or "butters" [spreads] made from them), cooked dried beans, and lean meats (taking care to limit highly processed high-sodium meats to once per week considering all meals).

Serving snacks to meet a weekly pattern Approaches to meet this requirement will need to be developed and tested to determine the most practical methods of implementation and monitoring.

Using the enhanced snack option If the enhanced snack is provided in place of two regular snacks, it will be expected to reduce the time required for serving and clean-up.

General Measures

Regardless of the exact nature of the new Meal Requirements that are put into effect by USDA, measures that will promote their successful implementation include (1) involving the family, community, and other key stakeholders and (2) training state agency staff and providers.

Involving the family, community, and other key stakeholders The value of parental involvement in nutrition in child care is evident in the study *Improving Nutrition and Physical Activity in Child Care: What Parents Recommend* (Benjamin et al., 2008). In this study, parents recommended an increase in fruits and vegetables and the provision of more healthful meals. The authors concluded, "This information may be used to create or modify interventions or policies and to help motivate parents to become advocates for change in child care" (p. 1907). Partnerships with older American and child care policy makers, adult and child organization advocacy groups, and individuals in the child and adult care environment will be a key ingredient in the successful implementation of the recommendations related to changes in the meal pattern for increasing consumption of whole grains and reducing solid fats, added sugars, and sodium.

Additional ways to involve stakeholders include the following:

- Forming broad-based advisory committees specific to the different care settings. Useful tasks include the development of implementation timelines in advance of the new requirements. These timelines can inform planning for menu revisions, training, and budgets so that all processes are in place when the new requirements are released.
- Forming local partnerships including relevant state agencies responsible for program administration; program providers; and other key stakeholders, such as representatives from state licensing organizations. In many states, the licensing organizations require that licensed child care providers follow requirements that are similar to or more stringent than the CACFP Meal Requirements— regardless of their participation in the federal food program.

Training of state agency staff, sponsors, and program providers Adequate training for state agency staff with responsibility for administration of the programs is important to ensure the fidelity of the implementation of the new Meal Requirements. Because state agencies play a key role in delivering training and technical assistance to sponsoring institutions and program providers, state agencies will need comprehensive training. The delivery of effective training for the CACFP providers is the most essential component of successful implementation. Steps could be taken to partner with the National

Institute of Food and Agriculture Expanded Food and Nutrition Education Program (EFNEP), which would be especially helpful in training for providers in day care homes and adult day care (see Appendix M). Further information on training appears in the section "Providing Technical Assistance."

Providing nutrition education   Culturally appropriate nutrition education can be a useful strategy for promoting behavior change and increasing the consumption of more healthful foods on the part of clients. It may also be useful in addressing parents' or guardians' concerns and beliefs that may be in conflict with the recommended Meal Requirements. The work of the National Food Service Management Institute (NFSMI) in cataloging the many research-based nutrition education publications can be leveraged for use in the various child and adult care program settings. See Appendix M for more information about the NFSMI and other nutrition education resources.

Phasing in Changes

By convening a panel of expert CACFP sponsors, providers, state administrators, CACFP associations (see Appendix M), and trainers, it is possible that USDA could identify a process for phasing in the essential elements with the goal of supporting the recommended Meal Requirements. Such a group could identify steps to take to gradually reach the goal of meeting the full set of recommendations. For example, instead of requiring that breakfast include lean meat or meat alternate three times per week and extra bread or other grain product on the other two days, initially the provider could be given a choice of whether to serve meat or meat alternates at all. Similarly, a method could be devised to ensure that a wide variety of vegetables would be served over the week, with limits on starchy vegetables, but without specifying the exact number of servings from each vegetable subgroup to be served.[1] Simplified "rules" developed from the proposed table of food specifications (Table 7-8) might be made more stringent every year or two. This would provide a mechanism for gradually serving a greater proportion of the grain products as whole grain-rich foods and reducing the use of foods that are high in solid fats, added sugars, and sodium.

Providing Technical Assistance

To achieve effective implementation of the recommended Meal Requirements in a cost-effective manner, technical assistance will be needed. The technical support must be comprehensive and adaptable to all program settings.

---

[1] The committee definitely does not favor reducing the amount of vegetables required per day even though that would be the most effective cost-saving measure. See the section "Controlling Costs."

The recommended Meal Requirements involve major shifts in the current approach to managing the food service operation. Therefore, regardless of the approach being used by a day care facility, providers will need to learn specific strategies for meeting new Meal Requirements. The approaches will need to be tailored to the type of care facility. Among the many skills and competencies needed are culturally sensitive menu planning approaches, label reading, best practices for menu compliance, food purchasing and preparation techniques, controlling costs, relationships among nutrition and health, developmentally appropriate feeding practices, and keeping food safe to eat.

Training could include the use of step-by-step instructional materials—print, video, or web-based—and guided hands-on experiences. Many resources are available that USDA could tap to assist with developing training materials and/or provide the training. Some of these are listed in Appendix M. The following subsections highlight four types of technical assistance that will be needed as a result of changes in the Meal Requirements: (1) engaging stakeholders, (2) meeting menu planning challenges, (3) controlling costs, and (4) meeting reporting requirements.

Engaging Stakeholders

Because the recommended Meal Requirements call for substantial changes in meals served in CACFP care settings, there is a strong need to engage stakeholders and promote their acceptance and support of the changes. Providers, program participants, and family members are among the key stakeholders. Importantly, program providers will need support to become accepting of the new meal patterns and food specifications. Technical assistance will be needed for state agencies, sponsoring institutions, centers, and day care homes to develop the attitudes and skills needed to engage stakeholders in a way that gains their support of the changes.

Meeting Menu Planning Challenges

The recommended Meal Requirements pose new challenges that will require menu planners to approach their task with a clear understanding of the meal patterns and food specifications. Practical methods will need to be developed and tested to help providers meet a number of anticipated menu planning challenges specific to CACFP, such as the following:

- Increasing the amount of vegetables served daily, the daily proportion of grain foods that are whole grain-rich, and the variety of vegetables served over the day and week;
- Designing and grouping menu item choices to ensure that each child and adult receives meals that meet the minimum amounts of each food group and subgroup during the week;

- Providing the recommended variety of food groups in the snacks served over the week;
- Identifying food products in the local marketplace that are affordable, fit with the food specifications, and appeal to the CACFP participants;
- Implementing incremental menu item changes (to permit providers to develop the skills and abilities to prepare and serve the new items successfully); and
- Adapting menus to meet cultural preferences for vegetarians, and for accommodating food allergies, food intolerances, and specific dietary restrictions.

One priority is collaboration between USDA and state agencies responsible for program administration to revise related menu planning guidance materials, including the current *Food Buying Guide for Child Nutrition Programs* (USDA/FNS, 2008), to make its content compatible with the recommended Meal Requirements for both children and adults. To meet the meal pattern for each age group, program providers may benefit from learning to design cycle menus.[2] Cycle menus offer ease and clarity in counting the number and type of required fruits, vegetables, and grains for the week (thus helping providers to comply with meal pattern requirements). Cycle menus also may aid budgeting, purchasing (shopping), the preparation and service of new menu items, and overall meal quality. The sample menus that the committee wrote to illustrate the application of the standards for menu planning (see Appendix K) provide examples of sound principles of menu planning. However, they are not expected to be suitable for any particular CACFP setting without some adaptation for ethnic, cultural, and local food preferences; food availability; and the capabilities of the food service operation. CACFP providers may want to use these menus as guides when developing and tailoring their own specific menus.

Controlling Costs

Increasing the amount and quality of food to be consistent with the recommended Meal Requirements will increase food costs, as described in Chapter 8. USDA and Congress will need to determine the extent to which they will support the recommended Meal Requirements (and thus national initiatives to increase access to more healthful meals) through regulations or adequate funding, respectively. Substantial improvements

---

[2]The committee recognizes that currently some states do not allow the use of cycle menus.

in CACFP meals can be expected only to the extent that care providers (1) are mandated to provide more fruits and vegetables, a greater proportion of whole grain-rich grain foods, and *lean* meats or meat alternates rather than high-fat choices and (2) receive sufficient funding to make this possible. An unfunded mandate would be expected to result in a loss of CACFP providers. Increasingly, more state regulatory agencies are implementing policy changes to improve the healthfulness of meals served in licensed facilities. Making CACFP regulations and funding more congruent with these policies and with national initiatives to improve diet and health will foster better care for the vulnerable populations that require care.

The committee was asked to be sensitive to cost but not to make funding recommendations. The committee worked to address the needs of the target populations and align its recommendations for Meal Requirements with updated dietary guidance and nutritional science as directed by the committee's statement of task (see "The Committee's Task," Chapter 1). Although reducing the amount of vegetables in the recommended Meal Requirements would lower the cost substantially, doing so would be contrary to the *Dietary Guidelines*, which put a strong emphasis on consuming more vegetables to promote health, and also contrary to the first key element of Meal Requirement Recommendation 2.

At current federal reimbursement levels, providers will be challenged to meet the anticipated increase in food costs and increases in non-food meal costs described in Chapter 8. In addition, CACFP sponsors and administering state agencies will have substantially increased labor costs related to training, technical assistance, and monitoring. According to a USDA report, "costs reported by sponsors on average were about 5 percent higher than allowable reimbursement amounts" (USDA/ERS, 2006, p. 1). Technical assistance and training will be needed to help providers meet the Meal Requirements while controlling the expected increases in costs, but increases in food costs will be unavoidable. Unlike school operations, CACFP care facilities do not generate program revenue from á la carte or catering sales and thus have no mechanism to generate income other than increasing the cost of care to the client—a serious limitation in view of the high proportion of low-income clients.

Guidance would be helpful for the small "mom and pop" child and adult care facilities, including day care homes that serve low-income families primarily and that rely on local small grocery stores—especially to providers who are new to CACFP. Such stores generally have higher food prices (Powell et al., 2007). Lessons could be learned from the experienced providers who have made arrangements to procure food through supermarkets, big box stores, or food buying clubs to help reduce food costs— including the strategies they use to store food safely.

Meeting Reporting Requirements

The changes in the Meal Requirements will call for a revision of the reporting requirements, as indicated below. Otherwise, one of the unintended consequences could be an increase in disallowed meals and snacks (that is, a loss of income resulting from the denial of claims for reimbursement for meals served because the various requirements appear not to have been met). Technical assistance will be needed to enable child and adult care directors and/or key food service personnel to meet those reporting requirements efficiently and accurately. Providers must be given timely information on the various federal, state, and local policies and regulations (e.g., record keeping including meal counting; how to document appropriately using food purchasing receipts; menus; and other records)—along with clear instructions on how to meet them.

Well-designed and well-executed technical assistance could add value even to the best-run child and adult care centers and home operations by enhancing providers' nutrition knowledge, menu planning, food preparation, and business record-keeping skills.

Revising Reporting Requirements and Monitoring Procedures for CACFP Meals

Reporting Requirements

As described in Chapter 2, many CACFP providers have difficulty meeting reporting requirements—that is, providing the data needed to document that the meals they serve are eligible for reimbursement. The recommended Meal Requirements would make it even more challenging to meet the current reporting requirements without the needed training, technical assistance, and revisions to the reporting requirements described above.

Monitoring Procedures

One aspect of the current monitoring of CACFP meals focuses on the meal components with the objective of making certain that reimbursement is warranted for the meals that were served. The overall objective of a revised approach to this aspect of the monitoring of CACFP meals could be to ensure their nutritional quality and consistency with the *Dietary Guidelines*. USDA could consider both a short-term approach to monitoring during the initial stage of implementation of the new Meal Requirements and a revised approach during the second stage, once implementation is well under way. Because unintended consequences may arise as a result of extensive changes in the Meal Requirements, another suggested key focus of monitoring is the identification of problems that may need to be addressed by the state agency or USDA—and also of any unexpected benefits that would provide evidence of the need for continued support of the program.

During the first stage, at least for the next several years, monitoring could be directed toward facilitating the transition to the new Meal Requirements. The initial approach might address a few elements at a time but occur on a frequent basis. The emphasis might be on examining progress in meeting the Meal Requirements (especially those related to fruits, vegetables, whole grain-rich foods, and the food specifications), identifying training needs for CACFP sponsors and providers, and providing needed technical assistance to improve the CACFP meals.

The subsequent approach to monitoring (the second stage) could continue to focus on gathering and using information to enhance the ability of providers to plan, prepare, and serve meals that are consistent with the new Meal Requirements. This second stage of monitoring could focus on documenting that planned menus and prepared meals are consistent with the recommended meal pattern (the first step in ensuring that meals that are counted or claimed for reimbursement are consistent with program requirements).

During both stages of monitoring, a variety of methods could be used to monitor how well the CACFP facilities have implemented the new Meal Requirements. For example, monitors could focus on whether CACFP facilities are offering only low-fat and fat-free milks, at least half of the grains as whole grain-rich products, and the required numbers and types of fruits and vegetables. This level of review could include menu review.

All this information could be used to (1) establish a baseline for CACFP food operations, (2) identify technical assistance needs, (3) prepare a plan, in cooperation with CACFP providers, for addressing these needs, and (4) monitor progress over time. In addition to focusing on planned menus and prepared meals, the assessment would address CACFP providers' access to vegetables, fruits, and whole grains and participants' acceptance of them.

RECOMMENDATIONS TO SUPPORT THE IMPLEMENTATION OF THE REVISED MEAL REQUIREMENTS

In order to bring the Meal Requirements into alignment with the best available guidance, consistent with the nutritional requirements of other programs of the Food and Nutrition Service, the committee makes the following implementation recommendations:

Implementation Strategy Recommendation 1: **USDA, working together with state agencies, and health and professional organizations should provide extensive technical assistance to implement the recommended**

Meal Requirements. Key aspects of new technical assistance to providers include measures to continuously improve menu planning (including variety in vegetable servings and snack offerings across the week), purchasing, food preparation, and record keeping (see the section "Providing Technical Assistance" for more detail). Such assistance will be essential to enable providers to meet the Meal Requirements while controlling cost and maintaining quality.

Implementation Strategy Recommendation 2: **USDA should work strategically with the CACFP administering state agencies, CACFP associations, and other stakeholders to reevaluate and streamline the systems for monitoring and reimbursing CACFP meals and snacks.** The CACFP National Professional Association and the Child and Adult Care Food Program Sponsor's Association would be key partners. Several aspects of the existing monitoring and reimbursement processes will need to be revised to enable states to efficiently administer the CACFP program with the new recommended Meal Requirements in place. The procedures would be expected to (1) focus on meeting relevant *Dietary Guidelines* and (2) provide information for continuous quality improvement and for mentoring program operators to assist in performance improvement. Among the challenges will be the development of practical methods for states to monitor for the meeting of weekly requirements and for minimizing providers' reporting requirements.

To prepare for successful implementation of the new requirements, USDA must provide for comprehensive training and technical support to the state administering agencies either directly or in cooperation with partners. Those agencies, in turn, need to ensure that the providers can receive the appropriate types of technical support. Figure 9-1 depicts the paths by which technical assistance related to various competencies and skills reaches providers. Note that state agencies and sponsoring institutions both have roles in improving the competencies and skills of providers. State administrators, local sponsors, and providers could collaborate and network with local education agencies, universities, and state early child care providers to develop training materials or participate in training.

Policies and systems are already in place in a number of parts of the country that could assist USDA in gradually rolling out the Meal Requirements in a manner that would support state agencies, sponsoring organizations, and providers. Because of the diverse program settings and providers, USDA is strongly encouraged to develop or make available effective tools that will assist CACFP providers to successfully implement the new Meal Requirements. Such tools include lists of allowable and unallowable food items, web-based training and menu-planning tools, portion-size charts and

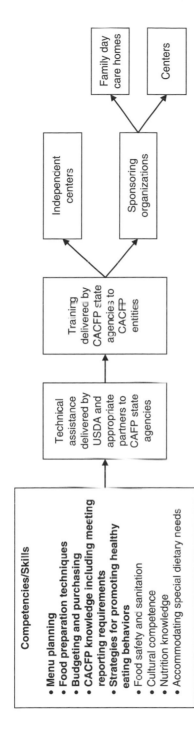

FIGURE 9-1 Paths for developing the competencies and skills of Child and Adult Care Food Program providers needed to implement recommended Meal Requirements.

NOTE: Current CACFP regulations require that state agencies as well as participating entities provide annual training to institutions and key staff. The competencies (in bold) are important areas for focus in order to achieve successful implementation of the revised Meal Requirements. However, competency is essential in all areas noted to ensure that healthy and safe meals and snacks are provided to program participants.

calculators, step-by-step calculators/charts to determine whole grain-rich food items, and lists of subgroups of vegetables. These tools must be sensitive to different cultures as well as geographic locations, and appropriate tools must be available for providers with language barriers or limited education.

The committee recognizes the NFSMI, EFNEP, and the USDA Agricultural Library (see Appendix M) as valuable starting places for information for all levels of key child and adult care personnel, but particularly for the directors and the food preparers. They provide excellent resources for networking, mentoring and training, and learning opportunities. Nonetheless, new resources will be needed to help providers meet the recommended Meal Requirements.

SUMMARY

Successful implementation of the recommended Meal Requirements will require attention to key elements of achieving change. The focus must be on providing extensive comprehensive technical assistance that is adapted for CACFP providers at all levels and on reevaluating and streamlining the systems for monitoring and reimbursing meals.

REFERENCES

Benjamin, S. E., J. Haines, S. C. Ball, and D. S. Ward. 2008. Improving nutrition and physical activity in child care: What parents recommend. *Journal of the American Dietetic Association* 108(11):1907–1911.

Bere, E., and K. I. Klepp. 2005. Changes in accessibility and preferences predict children's future fruit and vegetable intake. *International Journal of Behavioral Nutrition and Physical Activity* 2:15.

Birch, L. L. 1987. The role of experience in children's food acceptance patterns. *Journal of the American Dietetic Association* 87(9 Suppl):S36–S40.

Birch, L. L., and D. W. Marlin. 1982. I don't like it; I never tried it: Effects of exposure on two-year-old children's food preferences. *Appetite* 3(4):353–360.

Brug, J., N. I. Tak, S. J. te Velde, E. Bere, and I. de Bourdeaudhuij. 2008. Taste preferences, liking and other factors related to fruit and vegetable intakes among schoolchildren: Results from observational studies. *British Journal of Nutrition* 99(Suppl 1):S7–S14.

Burgess-Champoux, T., L. Marquart, Z. Vickers, and M. Reicks. 2006. Perceptions of children, parents, and teachers regarding whole-grain foods, and implications for a school-based intervention. *Journal of Nutrition Education and Behavior* 38(4):230–237.

Chan, H. W., T. Burgess-Champoux, M. Reicks, Z. Vickers, and L. Marquart. 2008. White whole-wheat flour can be partially substituted for refined-wheat flour in pizza crust in school meals without affecting consumption. *Journal of Child Nutrition and Management* 32(1). http://docs.schoolnutrition.org/newsroom/jcnm/08spring/en.asp (accessed October 6, 2010).

Cooke, L. 2007. The importance of exposure for healthy eating in childhood: A review. *Journal of Human Nutrition and Dietetics* 20(4):294–301.

Cullen, K. W., T. Baranowski, E. Owens, T. Marsh, L. Rittenberry, and C. De Moor. 2003. Availability, accessibility, and preferences for fruit, 100% fruit juice, and vegetables influence children's dietary behavior. *Health Education and Behavior* 30(5):615–626.

HHS/USDA (U.S. Department of Health and Human Services/U.S. Department of Agriculture). 2005. *Dietary Guidelines for Americans*, 6th ed. Washington, DC: U.S. Government Printing Office. http://www.health.gov/DietaryGuidelines/dga2005/document/ (accessed July 23, 2008).

IOM (Institute of Medicine). 2009. *The Public Health Effects of Food Deserts*. Washington, DC: The National Academies Press.

IOM. 2010. *Strategies to Reduce Sodium Intake in the United States*. Washington, DC: The National Academies Press.

Marquart, L. 2009. Incorporating Whole Grain Foods into School Meals and Snacks. Presented at the Institute of Medicine, Committee on Nutrition Standards for National School Lunch and Breakfast Programs Open Forum, Washington, DC, January 28, 2009.

Neumark-Sztainer, D., M. Wall, C. Perry, and M. Story. 2003. Correlates of fruit and vegetable intake among adolescents: Findings from Project EAT. *Preventive Medicine* 37(3):198–208.

Powell, L. M., S. Slater, D. Mirtcheva, Y. Bao, and F. J. Chaloupka. 2007. Food store availability and neighborhood characteristics in the United States. *Preventive Medicine* 44(3):189–195.

Rosen, R. A., L. Sadeghi, N. Schroeder, M. Reicks, and L. Marquart. 2008. Gradual incorporation of whole wheat flour into bread products for elementary school children improves whole grain intake. *Journal of Child Nutrition and Management* 32(1). http://www.schoolnutrition.org/Content.aspx?id=10584 (accessed October 6, 2010).

USDA/ERS (U.S. Department of Agriculture/Economic Research Service). 2006. *Administrative Costs in the Child and Adult Care Food Program: Reimbursement System for Sponsors of Family Child Care Homes*. http://ddr.nal.usda.gov/bitstream/10113/32789/1/CAT31012231.pdf (accessed October 12, 2010).

USDA/FNS (U.S. Department of Agriculture/Food and Nutrition Service). 2008. *Food Buying Guide for Child Nutrition Programs*. Alexandria, VA: USDA/FNS. http://teamnutrition.usda.gov/Resources/foodbuyingguide.html (accessed November 2, 2010).

Wardle, J., M. L. Herrera, L. Cooke, and E. L. Gibson. 2003. Modifying children's food preferences: The effects of exposure and reward on acceptance of an unfamiliar vegetable. *European Journal of Clinical Nutrition* 57(2):341–348.

10

Consistency of Recommendations for Meal Requirements and Implementation Strategies with the Committee's Criteria

The committee evaluated its recommendations for Meal Requirements for the Child and Adult Care Food Program (CACFP) and for the implementation of revised Meal Requirements using the criteria it established at the beginning of the study (see Chapter 6, Box 6-1). This chapter presents the committee's assessment of the consistency of these recommendations with the criteria.

OVERVIEW

The committee's criteria take into account the committee's task (stated in Chapter 1), an array of background information on the need for revisions to CACFP meal patterns, topics relevant to revising the current standards, and the critical areas for consideration provided to the committee by the U.S. Department of Agriculture (USDA) (see Appendix D). In developing recommendations for revised Meal Requirements and their implementation, the committee recognized that it is impossible to fully meet each of the criteria. Instead, it strived to find the best balance—Meal Requirements that would lead to appealing meals of high nutritional quality and that would be practical in a variety of settings and moderate in cost.

RECOMMENDATIONS FOR MEAL REQUIREMENTS ARE CONSISTENT WITH THE CRITERIA

The first three recommendations to USDA are for revisions to the current CACFP Meal Requirements. The primary goal of the recommended

Meal Requirements is to contribute to more healthful food and nutrient intakes by CACFP participants, especially in view of the high prevalence of obesity in the United States. As defined by the committee, the recommended Meal Requirements encompass both new meal patterns and new food specifications. The meal patterns are food-based targets that will promote intakes of healthy foods from five food groups: fruits, vegetables, low-fat dairy products, whole grains, and lean meats or meat alternates. The food specifications provide guidance on choices within these food groups that will lead to meals that have appropriate calorie levels and reduced amounts of solid fat, added sugars, and sodium. Although the impact of changes in the Meal Requirements on the daily food and nutrient intakes of CACFP participants cannot be predicted accurately, the recommended changes to the current Meal Requirements will likely improve the nutritional quality of the foods that are made available through the program. This, in turn, may have an indirect beneficial effect on food choices made outside the program, thus improving the overall nutritional status of participants.

Consistency of the Meal Requirement Recommendations with Criterion One

First Meal Requirement Recommendation

The first of the committee's recommendations addresses Meal Requirements for infants and young children:

USDA should adopt the recommended Meal Requirements for healthy infants up to 1 year of age.

This recommendation brings infant feeding recommendations into alignment with guidance from the American Academy of Pediatrics (AAP) and the Dietary Reference Intakes (DRIs), consistent with Criterion 1a.

Criterion 1: The Meal Requirements will be consistent with current dietary guidance and nutrition recommendations to promote health with the ultimate goal of improving participants' diets by reducing the prevalence of inadequate and excessive intakes of food, nutrients, and calories.

   a.   For infants and children younger than 2 years of age, the Meal Requirements will contribute to an overall diet that is consistent with established dietary recommendations for this age group and encourage and support breastfeeding for infants.

   b.   For participants ages 2 years and older, the Meal Requirements will be exemplified by the *Dietary Guidelines for Americans* and the Dietary Reference Intakes.

Key elements of the Meal Requirements appear below. (The meal patterns for this age group are presented in Chapter 7, Table 7-1.)

- Infants from birth to 6 months will be fed breast milk or formula exclusively.
- Infants ages 6–11 months will be fed breast milk or formula and appropriate solid foods.
- For infants ages 6–11 months, developmental readiness is to be considered in offering complementary foods.
- Infants from birth to 1 year will not be fed water or fruit juice.

The Meal Requirements for young children are also consistent with the DRIs. Meat and suitable meat alternates are emphasized for infants ages 6–11 months of age, to address concerns about iron and zinc intakes.

Although the committee was unable to develop strong incentives for breastfeeding through a mechanism related to the Meal Requirements, it encourages the development of such incentives. In addition, the recommendation to delay the introduction of solid foods until the infant is 6 months old is intended to encourage a longer period of full breastfeeding for breastfed infants.

Second Meal Requirement Recommendation

The second recommendation addresses variety and the quality of the foods served:

> For all children ages 1 year and older and for adults, USDA should adopt Meal Requirements that increase the variety of fruits and vegetables, increase the proportion of whole grains, and decrease the content of solid fats, added sugars, *trans* fats, and sodium (Tables 7-2 through 7-8).

This recommendation aligns adult and child feeding recommendations with the *Dietary Guidelines for Americans* and the DRIs, consistent with Criterion 1b, and recognizes that variety and diet quality are also important for younger children.

Alignment with guidance for 1-year-old children   The Meal Requirements for children 1 year of age were determined using three resources: AAP recommendations, MyPyramid food group recommendations for young children, and caloric and nutrient targets for children of this age. Although MyPyramid was not designed for children under 2 years of age, it was deemed to be an appropriate guide for setting meal patterns for 1-year-old children, with minor adjustments such as the use of whole milk rather than

---

BOX 10-1
Recommended Meal Requirements Improve
Alignment with *Dietary Guidelines*

- Better control of calories
- More fruits and vegetables
- A greater variety of vegetables
- More whole grain-rich foods, fewer refined grain foods
- Milk choices limited to nonfat and low-fat; no flavored milk for young children
- Increased emphasis on limiting foods high in solid fats and added sugars
- Minimized content of *trans* fat
- Stronger emphasis on gradual reduction of sodium

---

low-fat or nonfat milk. Thus, the amounts of food in the meal patterns provide young children who participate in CACFP with appropriate proportions of their daily nutrient needs, and Table 7-8 in Chapter 7 addresses appropriate food choices. Further information on the recommended Meal Requirements for 1-year-old children may be found in Chapter 7.

Alignment with the *Dietary Guidelines* The committee reviewed the recommended meal patterns for all age groups ages 2 years and older (Chapter 7, Tables 7-2 through 7-4), the food specifications (Chapter 7, Table 7-8), and the sample menus (Appendix K) to verify their correspondence with the *Dietary Guidelines*. It also determined the difference in the amounts of food in the current meal pattern with amounts in the recommended patterns (Chapter 8, Table 8-1). The recommended Meal Requirements clearly improve the alignment of CACFP meal patterns with the *Dietary Guidelines* (HHS/USDA, 2005). The amounts of fruits and vegetables are substantially higher in the new meal patterns for all these age groups, as is the proportion of whole grain-rich foods. In addition, milk products are the types encouraged in the *Dietary Guidelines*. The committee's review of the sample menus (Appendix K), which gave special attention to the inclusion of a variety of fruits and vegetables, whole grain-rich products, and nonfat or low-fat milk products, found that these menus are also consistent with the *Dietary Guidelines*. Box 10-1 highlights key ways in which the recommended Meal Requirements align with the *Dietary Guidelines*.

Examples of food specifications that show alignment with the *Dietary Guidelines* include the following:

- *Low-fat milk products*: Milk and yogurt will be nonfat or 1 percent fat; the use of low-fat cheese is encouraged.

- *Increasing the proportion of whole grains*: At least half of grain products must be whole grain-rich, and a higher proportion is encouraged.
- *Decreasing the intakes of saturated fat and added sugars*: Specifications limit milk fat and flavored milk; the only allowable form of juice is 100 percent juice with no added sugars; cereals are to contain less than 6 grams of sugar per ounce; and the frequency of use of high-fat meats and of grain foods high in solid fats and added sugars is limited.

As an example of how well the recommended meal patterns conform to the MyPyramid patterns (and thus to *Dietary Guidelines*), Table 10-1 shows a comparison of the recommended meal pattern to the MyPyramid pattern for preschool children ages 2–4 years, the largest age group that is currently served meals (rather than just snacks) by CACFP; similar tables for all age groups are shown in Appendix Tables J-4 through J-7. For children ages 2–4 years, the recommended meal pattern contains more fruit than the MyPyramid pattern and a smaller amount of vegetables. Although vegetables are not required at breakfast, they are allowed as a substitute for fruit, and it is likely that actual weekly menus will contain some vegetables. The amounts of grains, milk, and lean meat or meat alternates in the recommended pattern are very similar to those in the MyPyramid pattern.

Alignment with Dietary Reference Intakes To examine the alignment of the recommended Meal Requirements with the DRIs, the committee analyzed the sample breakfast and lunch menus for each age group using the Meals Menu Analysis program (see Appendix K in IOM, 2010, for a description of the program). The data are shown for children 2–4 years of age in Table 10-2, which compares the nutrients in the meal patterns with the daily nutrient targets by meal averaged over a 5-day week. Similar tables for all other age groups are shown in Appendix J, Tables J-8 through J-11. Notably, the sample menus meet or nearly meet the nutrient targets in almost all cases. Although calories appear to be somewhat low for all meals, additional calories will be provided by healthy fats and other fats and sugars that are permitted by the food specifications (e.g., the fat in 1 percent fat milk, and sugars in cereals and yogurt).

Based on analyses across all age groups, it appears prudent to make gradual changes to serve more foods that are rich in vitamin E and linoleic and α-linolenic acid (such as vegetable oils; nuts, seeds, and nut butters; and whole grains). The foods that are offered for this purpose need to be affordable, well accepted, and tolerated by CACFP participants (considering their age and physical abilities), and they need to fit within the calorie allowance. Although peanut butter is an example of a good source of vitamin E and the

TABLE 10-1 Comparison of MyPyramid Food Group Targets with MyPyramid Food Groups in Recommended Meal Patterns for Children 2–4 Years of Age

Food Group[c]	1,300-Calorie MyPyramid Pattern[a] for 2-4-Year-Olds[b] 1,300-kcal Daily MyPyramid Amts	1,300-kcal 5-Day Week[d] MyPyramid Amts	Weekly (5-Day) Allowance per Meal Breakfast 20%[e]	Pattern[f]	Lunch/Supper 26%	Pattern[f]	Snack 14%	Pattern[f]	5-Day Weekly Total[g]
Fruit (c)	1.25	6.25	1.25	2.5	1.63	2.5	0.88	1	9.5
Vegetables (c)	1.5	7.5	0	0	2.0	2.5	1.1	0.5	6
Dark green (c/wk)	1.5	1.1	0	0	0.28	0.5	0.15	0	1
Orange (c/wk)	1	0.7	0	0	0.19	0.5	0.10	0.25	1.5
Dry beans (c/wk)	1	0.7	0	0	0.19	0.25	0.10	0	0.5
Starchy (c/wk)	2.5	1.8	0	0	0.46	0.5	0.25	0	1
Other (c/wk)	4.5	3.2	0	0	0.84	0.75	0.45	0.25[h]	2
Grains (oz eq)	4.5	22.5	4.5	7	5.9	5	3.2	2	21
Meat and beans (oz eq)	3.5	17.5	3.5	3	4.6	5	2.5	2	17
Milk (c)	2	10	2.0	2.5	2.6	2.5	1.4	1	9.5

NOTES: Amts = amounts; c = cup; kcal = calories; oz eq = ounce equivalent; wk = week. The comparison of MyPyramid food group targets with the MyPyramid food groups in the recommended meal patterns for children ages 1 year, 5–13 years, 14–18 years, and adults are located in Appendix J, Tables J-4 through J-7. For consistency within the table, decimals, instead of fractions, are used in tables comparing MyPyramid pattern amounts and recommended CACFP 5-day meal patterns.

[a]1,300-calorie pattern based on an average of the 1,200- and 1,400-calorie patterns.

[b]Oil = 17 grams/day; discretionary calories = 171 kcal/day.

[c]See Appendix Table H-1 for a list of foods in the MyPyramid food groups and subgroups.

[d]Daily MyPyramid amounts multiplied by 5 to represent goals for a 5-day week.

[e]Proportional amount in each meal, based on the percent of calories in the meal; vegetables are not required at breakfast.

[f]Amounts in the meal pattern for each meal.

[g]Total MyPyramid amounts are calculated as follows: breakfast + lunch + supper + two snacks.

[h]The other vegetables served at snack are to be non-starchy vegetables only.

SOURCE: MyPyramid patterns from Britten et al., 2006.

TABLE 10-2 Comparison of Nutrients in Recommended Meal Patterns with Nutrient Targets Averaged Over a 5-Day Week for CACFP for Children 2–4 Years of Age

	Breakfast			Lunch/Supper			Snack		
	Nutr. Targets	Nutr. in Meals	% Diff.	Nutr. Targets	Nutr. in Meals	% Diff.	Nutr. Targets	Nutr. in Meals	% Diff.
Calories (kcal)	260	283	9	338	331	−2	182	142	−22
% Calories from fat	25–35	22	NA	25–35	26	NA	25–35	32	NA
% Calories from sat. fat	< 10	8	NA	< 10	9	NA	< 10	11	NA
Protein (g/d)	8.0	12	54	10	16	56	5.6	5.6	0
Vitamin A (µg RAE/d)	92	171	85	120	276	130	65	113	75
Vitamin C (mg/d)	15	18	21	20	28	41	11	7.5	−29
Vitamin E (mg αT/d)	1.4	0.40	−72	1.8	1.4	−24	1.0	0.49	−51
Thiamin (mg/d)	0.18	0.46	155	0.23	0.30	28	0.13	0.11	−13
Riboflavin (mg/d)	0.24	0.60	147	0.32	0.46	46	0.17	0.20	18
Niacin (mg/d)	2.4	4.7	101	3.1	4.0	31	1.6	1.3	−19
Vitamin B$_6$ (mg/d)	0.20	0.53	171	0.25	0.39	54	0.14	0.13	−5
Folate (µg DFE/d)	63	183	189	82	99	20	44	42	−5
Vitamin B$_{12}$ (µg/d)	0.56	1.6	186	0.72	1.1	45	0.39	0.44	13
Iron (mg/d)	1.7	4.6	172	2.2	2.5	12	1.2	1.0	−14
Magnesium (mg/d)	30	50	69	39	67	74	21	26	26
Zinc (mg/d)	1.3	2.7	119	1.6	2.3	42	0.88	0.89	2
Calcium (mg/d)	120	227	89	156	235	51	84	122	45
Phosphorus (mg/d)	167	261	56	217	304	40	117	129	11
Potassium (mg/d)	653	489	−25	849	656	−23	457	245	−46
Sodium (mg/d)	< 327	411	26	< 425	656	54	< 229	228	0
Linoleic acid (g/d)	1.6	0.96	−40	2.1	1.7	−19	1.1	0.85	−24
α-linolenic acid (g/d)	0.15	0.07	−54	0.20	0.19	−5	0.11	0.06	−44
Fiber (g/d)	4.2	3.3	−22	5.5	5.4	−2	2.9	1.7	−43

NOTE: αT = α-tocopherol; CACFP = Child and Adult Care Food Program; d = day; DFE = dietary folate equivalent; diff = difference; g = grams; kcal = calories; µg = micrograms; mg = milligrams; mo = month; NA = not applicable; nutr = nutrient; sat. fat = saturated fat; y = year.

unsaturated fatty acids, it is a food that many CACFP providers omit from meals because of concerns about nut allergies. The three nutrients that merit special attention—vitamin E, folate, and iron for meals served to children ages 12 years and older—are the same nutrients that were identified in the report *School Meals: Building Blocks for Healthy Children* (IOM, 2010).

Because no representative baseline menus were available, it was not possible to accurately determine changes in the nutrient content of menus based on the revised Meal Requirements. To obtain a rough estimate of the changes in nutrient content resulting from the modifications in requirements, however, the committee conducted an analysis using the baseline and revised food group composites (see Chapter 8 and Appendix I). The analysis specified differences in food take-up rates based on differences between current and recommended meal patterns. This crude analysis for children 2–4 years of age (see Table 10-3) shows that calories were slightly higher or the same as in the current meal patterns, but saturated fat decreased and most other nutrients increased at all the meals. Similar tables for all other age groups are shown in Appendix J, Tables J-12 through J-15.

Effects of nutrient intakes from CACFP meals on total daily nutrient intakes The analyses of the menu patterns (Chapter 7) and the recommended meal patterns (revised composites) (Table 10-2) and the comparison of revised composites with baseline composites (Table 10-3) all show that meals planned according to the recommended Meal Requirements, if they are consumed, have the potential to improve total daily nutrient intakes.

Consistency of the Meal Requirement Recommendations with Other Criteria

Recommendations 1 and 2 Regarding Meal Patterns and Food Specifications

Criterion 2 Both components of the recommended Meal Requirements—the meal patterns and the food specifications—contribute to meeting the goals specified in Criterion 2.

Criterion 2: The Meal Requirements will provide the basis for menus that are practical to plan, prepare, and serve in different settings.

The meal patterns allow choice from a wide range of foods, and the food specifications eliminate the need to count calories, saturated fat, or nutrients. State agencies would have the option of making food specifications

TABLE 10-3 Comparison of Nutrients at Baseline with Nutrients in Recommended Meal Patterns for Children 2–4 Years of Age

	Breakfast			Lunch/Supper			Snack		
	Baseline	Revised	% Change	Baseline	Revised	% Change	Baseline	Revised	% Change
Calories (kcal)	172	283	64	280	331	18	113	142	26
Fat (g)	4.7	7.0	50	12	9.6	-17	3.3	5.1	55
% Calories from Fat	24	22	-9	37	26	-30	26	32	23
Sat. fat (g)	2.4	2.5	4	4.8	3.2	-33	1.1	1.7	55
% Calories from sat. fat	13	8	-37	15	9	-43	9	11	23
Protein (g/d)	7.0	12	75	16	16	4	3.2	5.6	78
Vitamin A (µg RAE/d)	119	171	44	154	276	79	33	113	243
Vitamin C (mg/d)	14	18	34	11	28	162	9.8	7.5	-24
Vitamin E (mg αT/d)	0.28	0.40	43	0.76	1.4	84	0.27	0.49	81
Thiamin (mg/d)	0.18	0.46	156	0.24	0.30	25	0.09	0.11	22
Riboflavin (mg/d)	0.41	0.60	46	0.45	0.46	2	0.13	0.20	54
Niacin (mg/d)	1.4	4.7	236	3.1	4.0	31	0.94	1.3	41
Vitamin B_6 (mg/d)	0.24	0.53	121	0.27	0.39	44	0.10	0.13	30
Folate (µg DFE/d)	55	183	230	60	99	65	30	42	40
Vitamin B_{12} (µg/d)	1.0	1.6	59	1.2	1.1	-15	0.21	0.44	110
Iron (mg/d)	1.3	4.6	262	1.6	2.5	56	0.75	1.0	36
Magnesium (mg/d)	32	50	57	45	67	49	17	26	58
Zinc (mg/d)	1.1	2.7	151	2.1	2.3	8	0.45	0.89	98
Calcium (mg/d)	219	227	3	250	235	-6	64	122	92
Phosphorus (mg/d)	200	261	31	287	304	6	72	129	79
Potassium (mg/d)	410	489	19	504	656	30	180	245	36
Sodium (mg/d)	166	411	147	493	656	33	129	228	76
Linoleic acid (g/d)	0.43	0.96	123	1.4	1.7	21	0.58	0.85	47
α-linolenic acid (g/d)	0.07	0.07	0	0.16	0.19	19	0.05	0.06	20
Fiber (g/d)	1.7	3.3	98	2.4	5.4	122	1.1	1.7	53

NOTE: αT = α-tocopherol; CACFP = Child and Adult Care Food Program; d = day; DFE = dietary folate equivalent; g = grams; kcal = calories; µg = micrograms; mg = milligrams; mo = month; sat. fat = saturated fat; y = year.

easier to use by identifying lists of foods that need to be limited because of their content of solid fats, added sugars, and/or sodium.

Criterion 3 The meal patterns and food specifications that make up the Meal Requirements clearly provide the basis for incorporating nutritious foods and beverages, as specified in Criterion 3.

Criterion 3: The Meal Requirements will provide the basis for menus that incorporate healthful foods and beverages and are appealing to diverse age ranges and cultural backgrounds.

The choices within the five major food groups (meal components) allow for menus suitable for many different cultures. The sample menus in Chapter 7 and Appendix K follow the recommended Meal Requirements and are quite similar to menus that are used and well accepted in CACFP facilities in the southwestern United States. Nonetheless, the committee recognizes that a number of the recommended changes listed below will call for new measures (see Chapter 9) to increase the appeal of some of the foods:

- *Dark green and orange vegetables and legumes on the menu each week.* Few children and adults eat the amounts of vegetables recommended in MyPyramid (National Health and Nutrition Examination Survey [NHANES] 2003–2004; see Tables 4-1 and 5-1). Each vegetable subgroup includes many choices, however, and favorites from each group may be prepared in appealing ways.
- *More vegetables at lunch but starchy vegetables served less often.* Data from NHANES 2003–2004 indicate that vegetable consumption by children and adults is very low, with the exception of potato consumption (see Tables 4-1 and 5-1). However, the committee anticipates that parents and participants will ultimately appreciate the value of nutritionally improved CACFP meals and that, with repeated exposures, participants will learn to better appreciate the vegetable items offered (see the section "Implementing Key Elements for Clients Ages 1 Year and Older" in Chapter 9 for the basis of this expectation).
- *Milk choices limited to fat-free (plain or flavored) and plain low-fat (1 percent milk fat or less) for participants over 2 years of age.* Currently, a majority of American school-age children consume milk with a fat content of 2 percent or more, or flavored milk with at least 1 percent milk fat (USDA/FNS, 2008). Gradual reduction in the fat content of the milk may promote acceptance of the lower fat milks.

- *More whole grain-rich food products, fewer refined grain products.* Data from 2003–2004 (covered in Chapters 4 and 5) indicate that the consumption of whole grains by both children and adults is very low. This may be, in part, a function of the availability of suitable and appetizing whole grain foods. The committee anticipates that the availability of appealing and palatable whole grain products will increase with time.
- *Nearly all entrées, cheese, and grain products are low in saturated fat.* Modified recipes and training in food preparation can help make these foods more acceptable.
- *Minimal levels of* trans *fat in foods.* Although many processed foods still contain *trans* fat, added *trans* fats are being reduced or eliminated from the food supply. Little effect on the acceptability of these foods is expected.
- *Fewer desserts with meals.* Anecdotal evidence and evidence from Dillon and Lane (1989) indicate that desserts are very popular when served. They need to be limited, however, because they are a prominent source of solid fats, added sugars, and sodium and are typically low in nutrients and fiber.
- *Less sodium in meals.* High sodium intake is typical for U.S. children and adults. Modified recipes and training in food preparation and presentation can help providers reduce sodium in meals while retaining their appeal, but providers will need to depend to a large extent on sodium reductions by the food industry. For providers who can shop in stores large enough to offer a reasonable selection of foods, training in label reading may be very helpful. The reduction of the sodium content of CACFP meals is expected to be gradual.

The committee acknowledges the value of a gradual phase-in period to accustom participants to the changes in the menus and also to give the providers time to improve their skills for preparing and serving appealing meals according to the recommended Meal Requirements. The committee is optimistic that participants and providers will benefit from more healthful meals served at CACFP homes and centers and that, with effective implementation of the recommended Meal Requirements by providers, participants will find the meals appealing.

Criterion 4 The committee developed the Meal Requirements with providers in mind, as specified by Criterion 4.

Criterion 4: The Meal Requirements will facilitate the planning of menus that are compatible with the capabilities and resources for the variety of program providers.

The intent was to make the recommended Meal Requirements adaptable to different provider venues: day care homes, centers, and other facilities such as Head Start. However, in the short term, program providers in all these venues are likely to face challenges in obtaining acceptable products, especially whole grain-rich foods and foods that are reduced in solid fats, added sugars, and sodium. Changes in the types of food served, such as more fruits and vegetables, may increase preparation time and requirements for equipment and refrigeration. This is a particular concern for day care homes with small kitchens and limited resources (see Chapter 9).

Criterion 5 Throughout the process of developing the Meal Requirements, the committee kept cost in mind, as specified in Criterion 5.

Criterion 5: The Meal Requirements will allow the planning of menus that are sensitive to considerations of cost.

Nonetheless, revisions to the current Meal Requirements to improve alignment with *Dietary Guidelines* and the DRIs result in increased costs. In particular, as demonstrated in Chapter 8, increasing the amount of fruits, vegetables, and whole grain-rich foods in meals and snacks served by CACFP providers increases food costs. The expected increase will likely exceed the amount that can be absorbed by CACFP providers under current federal reimbursement levels.

Meal Requirement Recommendation 3 Regarding Enhanced Snack Option

The last of the recommendations for the Meal Requirements provides the option of an enhanced snack for adults and children 5 years of age and older:

> **USDA should give CACFP providers the option of serving one enhanced snack in the afternoon in place of a smaller snack in both the morning and the afternoon.**

This recommendation is particularly supportive of Criterion 2, to provide menus that incorporate healthful foods and beverages and are appealing to diverse age ranges and cultural backgrounds. The committee believes that an enhanced snack will be particularly appealing to older adults and to school-age children who participate in afterschool CACFP programs. The larger snack will also have the potential to add more healthful foods and beverages to the daily diet for those who may not consume a nutritious dinner and those who would otherwise consume less healthful snack items.

Because an enhanced snack provides more food items, it can be better tailored to cultural and other types of food preferences.

RECOMMENDATIONS FOR IMPLEMENTATION STRATEGIES ARE CONSISTENT WITH THE CRITERIA

First Implementation Recommendation

The first of the recommendations for implementation strategies addresses the need to help CACFP providers with the transition to the new Meal Requirements:

> USDA, working together with state agencies and health and professional organizations, should provide extensive technical assistance to CACFP providers to implement the recommended Meal Requirements.

This recommendation is particularly relevant to Criterion 3, which states that menus should be practical to plan, purchase, prepare, and serve in different settings. The committee recognizes that the recommended meal patterns are more complex than the current ones, especially because of the weekly requirements for vegetable subgroups and the requirement that at least half of the grains be whole grain-rich. In addition, limits on the frequency of use of foods high in solid fats and added sugars will call for careful attention to menu planning. Under the current requirements, the focus is simply providing minimum amounts of foods from four food components, and there is considerable leeway for offering extra menu items (such as condiments) and foods high in solid fats and added sugars. Technical assistance in the form of well-targeted training and new resource materials will be needed to equip CACFP providers to meet the menu planning challenges posed by the recommended Meal Requirements (see Chapter 9).

This implementation recommendation also supports Criterion 4, which focuses on providers' capabilities and resources. Providers in all venues will need training and other types of support to plan menus that meet the recommended Meal Requirements and that are realistic for their situation.

Second Implementation Recommendation

The second recommendation related to implementation strategies considers how providers and sponsors will be monitored and reimbursed:

> USDA should work strategically with the CACFP administering state agencies, CACFP associations, and other stakeholders to reevaluate and streamline the system for monitoring and reimbursing CACFP meals and snacks.

This recommendation is particularly relevant to Criterion 4, which addresses the capabilities and resources of program providers, and also to Criterion 5, which addresses cost. As discussed in Chapter 9, providers will need an easily followed revised reporting method to demonstrate that the meals they serve are eligible for reimbursement through CACFP. Furthermore, an efficient revised system for both monitoring and reimbursement will help control administrative costs.

SUMMARY

It is clear that the recommended Meal Requirements will result in menus that are more closely aligned with the *Dietary Guidelines* and the DRIs than are menus planned using the current meal requirements. In particular, the recommended Meal Requirements will provide more fruits and vegetables, a wider variety of vegetables, and a higher proportion of whole grain-rich foods while decreasing the offering of foods that are high in solid fats, added sugars, and sodium. However, these improvements in nutritional quality can be achieved only at somewhat higher cost and only if measures are taken to gain the support of providers, to develop some new skills, and to develop a streamlined system for monitoring and reimbursing CACFP meals and snacks. The committee anticipates that the recommended Meal Requirements are attainable with appropriate support for their implementation.

REFERENCES

Britten, P., K. Marcoe, S. Yamini, and C. Davis. 2006. Development of food intake patterns for the MyPyramid Food Guidance System. *Journal of Nutrition Education and Behavior* 38(6 Suppl):S92.

Dillon, M. S., and H. W. Lane. 1989. Evaluation of the offer vs. serve option within self-serve, choice menu lunch program at the elementary school level. *Journal of the American Dietetic Association* 89(12):1780–1785.

HHS/USDA (U.S. Department of Health and Human Services/U.S. Department of Agriculture). 2005. *Dietary Guidelines for Americans*, 6th ed. Washington, DC: U.S. Government Printing Office. http://www.health.gov/DietaryGuidelines/dga2005/document/ (accessed July 23, 2008).

IOM (Institute of Medicine). 2010. *School Meals: Building Blocks for Healthy Children*. Washington, DC: The National Academies Press.

USDA/FNS (U.S. Department of Agriculture/Food and Nutrition Service). 2008. *Diet Quality of American School-Age Children by School Lunch Participation Status: Data from the National Health and Nutrition Examination Survey, 1999–2004*. Alexandria, VA: USDA/FNS. http://www.fns.usda.gov/OANE/menu/published/CNP/FILES/NHANES-NSLP.pdf (accessed August 20, 2008).

11

Evaluation and Research Recommendations

The current meal requirements for Child and Adult Care Food Program (CACFP) participants have been in place since 1989. Implementing the recommendations for revisions to the CACFP meal requirements contained in this report would align the meals served with the *Dietary Guidelines for Americans* (HHS/USDA, 2005) and improve consistency with the food package provided by the U.S. Department of Agriculture (USDA) Supplemental Food Program for Women, Infants, and Children (WIC) (USDA/FNS, 2009) and with recommendations for school meals (IOM, 2010). A major change in the Meal Requirements in CACFP will have an impact on participants and program operators in a broad array of settings including child care centers and homes, adult care centers, emergency shelters, and afterschool programs. The following recommendations focus on a plan of ongoing evaluation, targeted research, and periodic reassessment to determine the magnitude of impact and identification of the need for future revisions in the Meal Requirements.

RECOMMENDATIONS FOR EVALUATION

Program Evaluation Recommendation 1: **USDA, in collaboration with relevant agencies, should provide support for research to evaluate the impact of the Meal Requirements on participants' total and program-related dietary intake and consumption patterns, on the food and nutrient content of the meals and snacks served, on demand from eligible providers to participate in CACFP, and on program access by participants.** This evaluation would determine (a) the food and nutrient content of meals and snacks as

183

served, (b) participant's overall food and nutrient intakes as related to current dietary guidance, and (c) the number of providers and participants in the CACFP program.

Program Evaluation Recommendation 2: **USDA should take appropriate actions to establish the current baselines prior to implementation of the new Meal Requirements for comparison purposes.** Collection of a nationally representative baseline database of foods actually served is crucial. It will also be important to collect information on significant factors that might influence the impact of CACFP, including the number and types of meals served by age and setting, variations in state licensing requirements, and differences in the cost of living. Comparing CACFP child care to non-CACFP child care in the same geographic location could also contribute to fully understanding the impact of CACFP.

Program Evaluation Recommendation 3: **To the extent possible, USDA should take steps to ensure that the final rule for the new Meal Requirements is informed by the results of evaluation of program impact** (described in Recommendation 1 above). It will be critically important to evaluate the extent to which implementation of the revised Meal Requirements achieves the goal of promoting health and improving participants' diets by reducing the prevalence of inadequate and excessive intakes of foods, nutrients, and calories, and contributing to an overall diet consistent with established dietary recommendations including the *Dietary Guidelines for Americans*. To gain a comprehensive understanding of this dynamic, the evaluation should determine the impact of the Meal Requirements on

- participants' total and program-related dietary intakes and consumption patterns,
- the food and nutrient content of the meals and snacks served,
- demand by child care and other eligible providers for the program, and
- access to the program by eligible participants.

Key Evaluation Components

Evaluate Impact of Meal Requirements

Evaluating the impact of the Meal Requirements on participant's total and program-related dietary intakes and consumption patterns requires consideration of the following components:

1. *Consistency with the* Dietary Guidelines for Americans:
    - What changes have occurred in the consumption by CACFP participants, through CACFP meals and snacks and overall,

of key food groups encouraged by the *Dietary Guidelines for Americans*, but often underconsumed, including fruits and vegetables, low-fat/fat-free milk products, and whole grain-rich foods?
- Do diets conform more closely to the *Dietary Guidelines*?
- How do participant's food group intakes compare with the daily dietary patterns recommended in the MyPyramid food guidance system?

2. *Nutrient Intakes*:
- What may be the effect of the recommended Meal Requirements on participant's nutrient intakes, both from meals and snacks served in care/program settings and across the day?
- Has the prevalence of inadequate or excessive nutrient intakes been improved?
- Do the Meal Requirement age-range categories function effectively?
- Were the desired mean (or range of) calorie intakes for each age group achieved?
- How did the distribution of energy intake per kilogram of body weight change?

3. *Participant Acceptance of Meals and Snacks*:
- Have the Meal Requirements allowed program operators to offer nutritious foods and beverages that are readily acceptable, widely available, commonly consumed, and appealing to participants of diverse cultural backgrounds?
- What is the feedback from participants regarding the desirability of the meals and snacks offered under the new Meal Requirements?
- Have the Meal Requirements changed the percentage of plate waste overall and for foods commonly underconsumed relative to the *Dietary Guidelines for Americans*?

Evaluating the impact of the Meal Requirements on the food and nutrient content of the meals and snacks served requires consideration of the following components:

4. *Food and Nutrient Content*:
- Do the meals and snacks served meet the Meal Requirements and the corresponding Target Median Intakes specified in this report?
- Are the meals and snacks served in CACFP consistent with the *Dietary Guidelines for Americans* and the Dietary Reference Intakes?

- What changes have occurred in the availability, through CACFP meals and snacks, of key food groups encouraged by the *Dietary Guidelines for Americans* but often underconsumed, including fruits and vegetables, low-fat/fat-free milk products, and whole grains?
- How do the foods offered in CACFP meals and snacks compare with the dietary patterns recommended in the MyPyramid food guidance system?
- What are the barriers and facilitators to providing meals and snacks to participants that meet the recommended Meal Requirements?

5. *Food Procurement, Preparation, and Service Patterns*:
   - Have the Meal Requirements been compatible with the development of menus that are practical to prepare and serve in a variety of different settings? If not, what aspect(s) of the Meal Requirements is/are incompatible, in what settings, and what adjustments are needed to address the issues identified?
   - Are the Meal Requirement age-range categories practical for program meal service operations?
   - What skills and technology do program operators need to operate within the new Meal Requirements effectively?
   - How do the changes in the Meal Requirements affect the time required by state agencies and sponsoring organizations monitoring institutions and facilities?
   - Is the expanded variety of recommended foods available in food markets accessed by providers?

Evaluating the impact of the Meal Requirements on the demand from eligible providers to participate in CACFP and on access by eligible participants requires consideration of the following components:

6. *Demand*:
   - Have the new Meal Requirements affected the demand for CACFP by program operators in child care and other settings?
   - What are the program operators' perceptions of participating in the program under the new Meal Requirements? Has this changed over time? Has this impacted word-of-mouth program endorsements?
   - Have the trends for CACFP participation rates of child care centers and homes, adult care centers, emergency shelters, and afterschool programs changed at the national, regional, and/or state level?

- Have the trends in the number of participants (children, teens, and/ or elderly) overall and specifically in child care centers and homes, adult care centers, emergency shelters, and afterschool programs changed at the national, regional, and/or state level? Have the saturation rates for these programs changed over time?
- Has the relative distribution of meal types changed within the range of program settings at the national, regional, and/ or state level?

7. *Factors Potentially Influencing Demand*:
   - How well have the projected costs compared to the actual costs of the recommended Meal Requirements, and how do costs vary by geographic location and setting?
   - What is the impact of the Meal Requirements on the reimbursement levels?
   - Does CACFP align with other USDA Child Nutrition and WIC programs, allowing a smooth interface for program operators and a consistent nutrition message for program participants and their families?

RECOMMENDATIONS FOR RESEARCH

Targeted Research

Research Recommendation 1: **USDA, in collaboration with relevant agencies and foundations, should support research on topics related to the implementation of the Meal Requirements and to fill important gaps in knowledge of the role of CACFP in meeting the nutritional needs of program participants.** This targeted research should including the following:

- What are the best ways to maximize the value of the new Meal Requirements in providing good nutrition for children and adults in the various CACFP settings? How can meal-time environmental factors be used in CACFP child care settings to help facilitate healthy eating?
  - What are the best practices to educate and engage staff, parents, guardians, and caregivers to fully support the new Meal Requirements?
  - How can CACFP play a more effective role in encouraging and supporting breastfeeding?
- How do environmental disparities in access to healthy food at affordable prices affect both demand for CACFP and the ability of program operators to meet CACFP Meal Requirements?
  - Does this affect the types and quality of foods offered through CACFP meals and snacks in food deserts?

○   Can CACFP participation under the new Meal Requirements increase the availability of affordable healthy foods in the grocery stores in a neighborhood?

•   How does participation in CACFP under the new Meal Requirements affect children and adult weight status, including the dynamics of obesity and its consequences; food insecurity, including the consequences of chronic food insecurity the connection between hunger and obesity; children's dietary intake and diet quality, including program impacts on household food expenditures, food purchases, food choices, and nutrient intake; and the trade-offs in balancing work, child care, and food preparation?

•   What nutrition and dietary guidelines are needed for infants and young children?

○   How can the *Dietary Guidelines* be extended to a coordinated set of recommendations for infants and young children?

Periodic Reassessment

A revision of the *Dietary Guidelines for Americans* is expected to be released in 2011, and further revisions of the *Dietary Guidelines* are expected at periodic intervals thereafter. Similarly, the DRIs for vitamin D and calcium currently are under review, and changes in the DRIs for various other nutrients may be published in the future. Furthermore, the American Academy of Pediatrics periodically updates its recommendations for infants and children. To keep the Meal Requirements aligned with these sources of dietary guidance, periodic review is necessary, followed by revisions if needed. The recent release of the report of the 2010 Dietary Guidelines Advisory Committee (USDA/HHS, 2010) provides an opportunity to suggest types of revision that might be needed.

The committee's reading of the advisory committee's preliminary report revealed a few proposed changes in dietary guidance that might affect the Meal Requirements. Most notably, that report presents a somewhat different set of vegetable subgroups, with changes in weekly recommended amounts of some subgroups. If adopted as policy, the change would call for the Meal Requirements to adopt the vegetable subgroup revisions and to make small adjustments in the recommended number of servings of vegetable subgroups over the week. The advisory committee's proposed lowering of the values for maximum sodium and saturated fat intakes, if adopted, might eventually call for somewhat stricter food specifications.

Research Recommendation 2: **USDA should review and update, as appropriate, the CACFP Meal Requirements to maintain consistency with the *Dietary Guidelines* and other relevant science.** Periodic reassessment of the program meal requirements should be undertaken to ensure that the meals and snacks served

- Are consistent with the goals of the most recent *Dietary Guidelines for Americans* and
- Promote the health of the population served by the program as indicated by the most recent relevant nutrition science.

This process should include a review of costs to program operators resulting from updated requirements for meals and snacks served under the program.

SUMMARY

The effect of the recommended Meal Requirements for CACFP should be examined through an initial short-term evaluation as well as through ongoing periodic evaluations. Targeted research is needed to fill important gaps in our knowledge of the nutritional needs of CACFP recipients. Periodic reassessment of the Meal Requirements is needed to ensure consistency with the latest dietary guidance. Funding will be needed to support these research and evaluation activities.

REFERENCES

HHS/USDA (U.S. Department of Health and Human Services/U.S. Department of Agriculture). 2005. *Dietary Guidelines for Americans*, 6th ed. Washington, DC: U.S. Government Printing Office. http://www.health.gov/DietaryGuidelines/dga2005/document/ (accessed July 23, 2008).

IOM (Institute of Medicine). 2010. *School Meals: Building Blocks for Healthy Children*. Washington, DC: The National Academies Press.

USDA/FNS (U.S. Department of Agriculture/Food and Nutrition Service). 2009. *Women, Infants, and Children*. http://www.fns.usda.gov/wic/ (accessed March 24, 2010).

USDA/HHS (U.S. Department of Agriculture/U.S. Department of Health and Human Services). 2010. *Report of the Dietary Guidelines Advisory Committee on the Dietary Guidelines for Americans, 2010*. http://www.cnpp.usda.gov/DGAs2010-DGACReport.htm (accessed June 29, 2010).

A

Acronyms, Abbreviations, and Glossary

ACRONYMS AND ABBREVIATIONS

AAP	American Academy of Pediatrics
ADA	American Dietetic Association
AI	Adequate Intake
αT	α-tocopherol
AMDR	Acceptable Macronutrient Distribution Range
AoA	Administration on Aging
ARS	Agricultural Research Service, U.S. Department of Agriculture
BMI	body mass index
BRFSS	Behavioral Risk Factor Surveillance System
c	cup
CACFP	Child and Adult Care Food Program
CDC	Centers for Disease Control and Prevention
CFR	Code of Federal Regulations
CI	confidence interval
CNPP	Center for Nutrition Policy and Promotion, U.S. Department of Agriculture
CSFII	Continuing Survey of Food Intakes by Individuals
DFE	dietary folate equivalent
DGA	*Dietary Guidelines for Americans*

DRI   Dietary Reference Intakes

EAR   Estimated Average Requirement
EER   Estimated Energy Requirement
EFNEP   Expanded Food and Nutrition Education Program
eq   equivalent
ERS   Economic Research Service, U.S. Department
         of Agriculture

FCS   Food and Consumer Service, U.S. Department
         of Agriculture
FDA   Food and Drug Administration
FFVP   Fresh Fruit and Vegetable Program
FITS   Feeding Infants and Toddlers Study
fl   fluid
FNDDS   Food and Nutrient Database for Dietary Studies
FNS   Food and Nutrition Service, U.S. Department of
         Agriculture
FY   fiscal year

g   gram

HHS   U.S. Department of Health and Human Services

IOM   Institute of Medicine, The National Academies
IU   international unit

kcal   kilocalorie/calorie
kg   kilogram

mg   milligram
MPED   MyPyramid Equivalents Database

NCHS   National Center for Health Statistics, CDC
NFSMI   National Food Service Management Institute
NHANES   National Health and Nutrition Examination Survey
NIH   National Institutes of Health
NRC   National Research Council, The National Academies
NSLP   National School Lunch Program

OR   odds ratio
oz   ounce

| PAL | physical activity level |
| P.L. | Public Law |

RA/RAE	retinol activity/retinol activity equivalent
RDA	Recommended Dietary Allowance
RNI	Recommended Nutrient Intakes

| SBP | School Breakfast Program |
| SoFAS | solid fats and added sugars |

T	tablespoon
TMI	Target Median Intake
tsp	teaspoon

µg	microgram
UL	Tolerable Upper Intake Level
USDA	U.S. Department of Agriculture

| WIC | Special Supplemental Nutrition Program for Women, Infants, and Children |

| y | years |

GLOSSARY

Acceptable Macronutrient Distribution Ranges The range of intakes of an energy source that is associated with a reduced risk of chronic disease yet that can provide adequate amounts of essential nutrients.

Adequate Intake A recommended average daily nutrient intake level based on observed or experimentally determined approximations or estimates of nutrient intake by a group or groups of apparently healthy people that are assumed to be adequate.

Composite Food Items 133 food item groupings, each of which represents several of many similar food items (for example, orange juice, which also includes lemon juice and lime juice). Based on research done by Marcoe et al. (2006)[1] in the development of the MyPyramid food guidance system. Also called "food clusters."

---

[1]Marcoe, K. W. Juan, S. Yamini, A. Carlson, and P. Britten. 2006. Development of food group composites and nutrient profiles for the MyPyramid food guidance system. *Journal of Nutrition Education and Behavior* 38(6 Suppl):S93–S107.

Dietary Reference Intakes A family of nutrient reference values established by the Institute of Medicine.

Enhanced Snack A single afternoon snack option for adults and children at least 5 years of age to be served in place of a smaller snack in both the morning and the afternoon. The enhanced snack would have the same requirements as two of the smaller snacks.

Estimated Average Requirement The usual daily intake level that is estimated to meet the requirement of half the healthy individuals in a life-stage and gender group.

Estimated Energy Requirement The average dietary energy intake that is predicted to maintain energy balance in a healthy adult of a defined age, weight, height, and activity level consistent with good health. In children and pregnant and lactating women, it includes the needs associated with deposition of tissues or the secretion of milk at rates consistent with good health.

Food Clusters See Composite Food Items.

Food Deserts Neighborhoods and communities that have limited access to affordable and nutritious foods.

Food Group One of five food groups that comprise reimbursable meals for children ages 1 year or older and adults planned to meet the meal requirements. The five food components are meat and meat alternate, grains and breads, fruits, vegetables, and fluid milk.

Food Specifications A phrase that indicates the types of infant foods and foods from the five food groups that will help achieve nutritional quality. In general, specifications help to limit foods that are high in solid fats, added sugars, and *trans* fat.

Meal Patterns A phrase used to refer to specified food groups and amounts to serve from each group for various age groups to achieve the meal requirements.

Meal Requirements A set of standards that encompasses two distinct elements: meal patterns and food specifications to be used for menu planning.

Menu Item Any single food or combination of foods, except condiments, served in a meal. All menu items or foods offered as part of the reimbursable meal will be counted toward meeting the Meal Requirements.

National School Lunch Program The program under which participating schools operate a nonprofit lunch program, in accordance with 7 C.F.R. Part 210.

Nutrient Density (of foods) The amount of a specific nutrient in a food per 100 calories of that food.

Nutrient Targets New recommended goals for the amounts of nutrients and other dietary components to be provided by CACFP meals. Nutrient Targets provide the scientific basis for developing Meal Patterns.

Reimbursable Meal A meal that (1) meets the standards set by the U.S. Department of Agriculture and (2) is served to an eligible participant. Such meals qualify for reimbursement with federal funds.

Representative Menus Menus from foods used by CACFP family day care providers that were selected using the CACFP component serving data for use in comparing nutrients and costs under the current Meal Requirements with those under the recommended Meal Requirements.

School Breakfast Program The program under which participating schools operate a nonprofit breakfast program in accordance with 7 C.F.R. Part 220.

Sponsoring Organization Organizations that enter into agreements with their administering state agencies to assume administrative and financial responsibility for CACFP operations.

State Agency Agencies within the states that administer the CACFP. In most states the state educational agency administers CACFP but in a few states it is administered by an alternate agency, such as the state health or social services department. The child care component and the adult day care component of CACFP may be administered by different agencies within a state, at the discretion of the governor.

Target Median Intake Statistically derived target for the median intake of a nutrient to be used to plan diets for groups.

Tolerable Upper Intake Level The highest daily nutrient intake level that is likely to pose no risk of adverse health effects to almost all individuals in the general population.

Usual Nutrient Intake Distribution A distribution of reported nutrient intakes based on 24-hour recalls, that has been statistically adjusted to better estimate a usual intake distribution; for this report, references to nutrient intake include intakes of energy (calories).

B

Biographical Sketches of Committee Members

SUZANNE P. MURPHY, Ph.D., R.D. (*Chair*), is a Researcher and Professor at the Cancer Research Center of Hawaii at the University of Hawaii, and director of the Nutrition Support Shared Resource at the center. Dr. Murphy's research interests include dietary assessment methodology, development of food composition databases, and nutritional epidemiology of chronic diseases (with emphasis on cancer and obesity). Dr. Murphy has served as a member of the National Nutrition Monitoring Advisory Council and the year 2000 Dietary Guidelines Advisory Committee. Currently, she serves on the editorial board for *Nutrition Today* and is a contributing editor for *Nutrition Reviews*. She is a member of various professional organizations including the American Dietetic Association, the American Society for Nutrition, the American Public Health Association, the Society for Nutrition Education, and the Society for Epidemiological Research. Dr. Murphy has served on several Institute of Medicine panels including the Committee on Nutrition Standards for National School Lunch and Breakfast Programs, the Subcommittee on Interpretation and Uses of Dietary Reference Intakes (as chair, then member); the Subcommittee on Upper Safe Reference Levels of Nutrients (as member); and the Panel on Calcium and Related Nutrients (as member). She chaired the Committee to Review the WIC Food Packages and is a member of the Food and Nutrition Board. Dr. Murphy earned an M.S. in molecular biology from San Francisco State University, and a Ph.D. in nutrition from the University of California-Berkeley. She is a registered dietitian.

NORMA D. BIRCKHEAD, B.S., is Manager of the Child and Adult Care Food Program (CACFP) for the Office of the State Superintendent of Education for the District of Columbia Government. Prior to this, she worked on CACFP at the federal level for the U.S. Department of Agriculture's Child Nutrition Division in the Child and Adult Care and Summer Food Service Programs Section. She currently provides operational support to staff with her nearly 30 years of extensive child and adult care and summer food service program knowledge and experience. She is responsible for the overall oversight, administration, management, and compliance for the District of Columbia's CACFP. In her role as manager of programs, she applies analytical techniques for developing new and modifying existing program operations, evaluates local program operations for adherence to federal requirements through analysis of data reporting, and identifies defects in the organizations' internal procedures and resolves discrepancies which may lead to failure to comply with program regulations. Ms. Birckhead earned her B.S. in elementary education from the District of Columbia Teacher's College, and she has completed some graduate work in organization behavior at Trinity College in Washington, DC.

ALICIA L. CARRIQUIRY, Ph.D., is Professor of Statistics at Iowa State University (ISU). Her research interests include Bayesian statistics and general methods. Her recent work focuses on nutrition and dietary assessment, as well as on problems in genomics, forensic sciences, and traffic safety. Dr. Carriquiry is an elected member of the International Statistical Institute (ISI), a Fellow of the Institute of Mathematical Statistics, and a Fellow of the American Statistical Association. She is Vice President of the American Statistical Association and a member of the Council of the International Statistical Institute. She has served on the Executive Committee of the Institute of Mathematical Statistics and has been a member of the Board of Trustees of the National Institute of Statistical Sciences. She is also past president of the International Society for Bayesian Analysis and a past member of the Board of the Plant Sciences Institute at ISU. Dr. Carriquiry is editor of *Statistical Sciences* and Associate Editor of *The Annals of Applied Statistics* and the Editor of the *Electronic Encyclopedia of Statistics* representing the ISI. She also serves on the editorial boards of several Latin American journals of statistics and mathematics. She currently serves or has previously served on several National Academy of Sciences committees, including the standing Committee on National Statistics, the Committee on Social Science Evidence for Use (2008–2009), the Committee on Gender Differences in Careers of Science, Engineering, and Mathematics Faculty (2004–2009), the Committee on Assessing the Feasibility, Accuracy, and the Technical Capability of a National Ballistics Database (2004–2008), the Committee on Applied and Theoretical Statistics (2003–2006), the Subcommittee on Use of Third Party Toxicity Research with Human Test Subjects (2002–2004), the Committee on Evaluation of USDA's Methodology for Estimating Eligibility and Participation for the WIC Program (2000–2003), and the Subcommittee on Interpretation and Uses of Dietary Reference Intakes (1998–2003). Dr. Carriquiry received her Ph.D. in statistics and animal genetics from ISU.

RONNI CHERNOFF, Ph.D., R.D., FADA, CSG, is the Director of the Arkansas Geriatric Education Center, Associate Director of the Geriatric Research, Education & Clinical Center for Education and Evaluation for the Central Arkansas Veterans Affairs Health System, and Professor of Geriatrics at the University of Arkansas for Medical Sciences. She is past president of the American Dietetic Association, where she also served as Chair of the Council on Research and Chair of the Commission on Dietetic Registration. Dr. Chernoff has published numerous abstracts, journal articles, and book chapters and is editor of the text, *Geriatric Nutrition: The Health Professional's Handbook*, Third Edition (2006). She has served as Editor-in-Chief of *Perspectives in Applied Nutrition*, as editor of *The Digest*, on the Editorial Boards of the *Journal of Parenteral and Enteral Nutrition* and the *Journal of the American Dietetic Association*, Associate Editor of *Nutrition in Clinical Practice*, and section co-editor for *Current Opinions in Clinical Nutrition*. She also served on the editorial boards of *Topics in Geriatric Rehabilitation, Nutrition Support Services, Clinical Management Newsletter, Directions in Clinical Nutrition, Senior Patient (Postgraduate Medicine)*, and the *Journal of Nutrition for the Elderly*. Her primary research interests are nutrition and aging and health promotion. Dr. Chernoff received her Ph.D. from the University of Pennsylvania.

SONIA COTTO-MORENO, M.P.H., R.D., L.D., is the Child Care Food Program Director for the Teaching and Mentoring Communities' (TMC) Migrant Seasonal Head Start Program. TMC is a private nonprofit super grantee providing comprehensive services to migrant children in seven states. She oversees CACFP and nutrition services for nearly 8,000 children from birth to compulsory school age. She consults regularly with peers from a variety of fields to help identify wellness activities to impact children and adults affected by the obesity epidemic. Ms. Cotto-Moreno has a Certificate of Child and Adult Weight Management from the American Dietetic Association and the Program for Infant and Toddler Caregivers. She currently serves on the TexAn Coalition in Texas, a group that was instrumental in developing the Strategic Plan for the Prevention of Obesity in Texas 2005–2010. She has been asked to share her expertise in communicating Hispanic nutrition-related health issues and a process for advocating with governing bodies on funding health initiatives, that is, physical activity and nutrition education curriculum to address obesity in Head Start programs. Ms. Cotto-Moreno was recently appointed to the Texas State Evaluation Council on Nutrition, Physical Activity and Obesity Prevention. She has written articles for the National Child Care Information Center and National Head Start Association (NHSA) magazines, and her advocacy for physical activity in Head Start has been documented by Washington Productions, Inc. She received her B.S. in dietetics from the University of Texas at Austin, and she completed her practicum experience compiling migrant programs' implementation plans for the Office of Head Start's physical activity initiative "I am Moving, I am Learning" in fulfillment of her M.P.H. in public health leadership at the University of North Carolina at Chapel Hill.

KAREN WEBER CULLEN, Dr.P.H., R.D., is Associate Professor of Pediatrics at the USDA/Agricultural Research Services (ARS) Children's Nutrition Research Center, Baylor College of Medicine. Her primary research interest is prevention of obesity and diet-related chronic diseases. Her current research includes exploration of strategies to increase school breakfast consumption in middle schools; development and evaluation of a website on healthy eating and physical activity for high school students; evaluation of a web-based program on healthy eating for African-American families; and dissemination of a video intervention on improving the family home food environment and food parenting tips for Cooperative Extension Expanded Food and Nutrition Education Program classes. Dr. Cullen recently served as a member of the IOM's Committee on Nutrition Standards for National School Lunch and Breakfast Programs. Dr. Cullen's professional memberships include the Society for Nutrition Education, the Society for Behavioral Medicine, the American Dietetic Association, and the Texas Dietetic Association (Distinguished Scientist Award in 2001). She is a member of the Dannon Institute Scientific Council, the Dannon Institute Schools Committee, and the Schools Committee of the Alliance for a Healthier Generation. Dr. Cullen has a M.S. in nutrition from Case Western Reserve University and a Dr.P.H. in health promotion and health education from The University of Texas School of Public Health.

MARY KAY FOX, M.Ed., is Senior Researcher and area leader for nutrition research at Mathematica Policy Research, Inc. Ms. Fox has more than 20 years of research experience with child nutrition and food assistance programs. She has conducted research on the adequacy and quality of diets consumed by children, from birth through adolescence, and has examined the contributions of school- and child care-based meal programs to children's dietary intakes and obesity risk. Ms. Fox led the nutrition components of two comprehensive national studies of CACFP and served as a co-principal investigator on the 2002 and 2008 Feeding Infants and Toddler Studies. She also assessed the implementation of an obesity prevention initiative in Head Start centers, including assessments of the types and quality of foods offered and opportunities for physical activity. Her awards include a distinguished service award from the American Dietetic Association and Recognized Young Dietitian of the Year from the Massachusetts Dietetic Association. She served on the IOM Committee on Nutrition Standards for National School Lunch and Breakfast Programs. Ms. Fox has a B.S. in nutrition and dietetics from Mundelein College of Loyola University and an M.Ed. in nutrition from Tufts University.

GERALDINE HENCHY, M.P.H., R.D., is Director of Nutrition Policy and Early Childhood Programs at the Food Research and Action Center. Ms. Henchy's focus is on CACFP and the Special Supplemental Nutrition Program for Women, Infants, and Children (WIC). She recently completed a national environmental scan of effective best practices and strategies for implementing enhanced nutrition standards and policies in CACFP. Ms. Henchy serves on the U.S. Department of Agriculture's CACFP Management Improvement Task Force, and she previously served as the consumer member on the U.S. Department of Agriculture's Advisory Board. She has been honored to receive awards for her work on CACFP from the Sponsors Association, the National Sponsors Forum, and the California Child Care Food Program Roundtable. Most recently, the National Association of Family Child Care honored Ms. Henchy with their Advocate of the Year Award. Ms. Henchy was a reviewer for the IOM report *Proposed Criteria for Selecting the WIC Food Packages*. Ms. Henchy is a founding member of the American Dietetic Association's Hunger and Malnutrition Practice Group (now the HEN practice group) and a past chair. She is a registered dietitian and has an M.P.H. in nutrition from the University of California, Berkeley.

HELEN H. JENSEN, Ph.D., is Professor in the Department of Economics, College of Agriculture and Life Sciences, at Iowa State University (ISU) and serves as Head of the Food and Nutrition Policy Division in the Center for Agricultural and Rural Development at ISU. Dr. Jensen's research concerns food demand and consumption, food assistance and nutrition policies, food security, and the economics of food safety and hazard control. She has been a member of the Board of Directors of the Agricultural and Applied Economics Association and the American Council on Consumer Interests, and she has served on the editorial boards of a number of professional journals. Dr. Jensen has previously served on several National Academies committees, including the IOM Committee to Review the WIC Food Packages and the Committee on Nutrition Standards for the National School

Lunch and School Breakfast Programs. She also served on the National Research Council's (NRC's) Committee on the Economic Development and Current Status of the Sheep Industry in the United States; the Committee on Assessing the Nation's Framework for Addressing Animal Diseases; the Committee on Biological Threats to Agricultural Plants and Animals; the Board on Agriculture's Panel on Animal Health and Veterinary Medicine; and the Committee on National Statistics' (CNSTAT) Panel to Review USDA's Measurement of Food Insecurity and Hunger. She currently serves as a member of the National Research Council's (NRC's) Committee on Ranking FDA Product Categories Based on Health Consequences, and as a member of the World Health Organization Initiative to Estimate the Global Burden of Foodborne Diseases, Foodborne Disease Burden Epidemiology Reference Group. Dr. Jensen holds an M.S. in agricultural and applied economics from the University of Minnesota, and a Ph.D. in agricultural economics from the University of Wisconsin-Madison.

CHARLENE RUSSELL-TUCKER, M.S.M., R.D., is Associate Commissioner for the Connecticut State Department of Education. In this role she is responsible for the administration of the Division of Family and Student Support Services, which comprises three bureaus: the Bureau of Choice Programs; the Bureau of Health/Nutrition, Family Services and Adult Education; and the Bureau of Special Education. She provides leadership and support in developing and implementing effective family and student support programs and services to assist schools and other educational partners in improving student performance. Prior to her appointment as Associate Commissioner, Ms. Russell-Tucker was Chief of the Bureau of Health and Nutrition Services and Child/Family/School Partnerships at the Connecticut State Department of Education. The Bureau was strategically positioned within the Department to support the social, emotional, physical, and mental health of students and families in order to achieve success in school and in life. Its initiatives and services include School-Family-Community Partnerships, Child Nutrition Programs, School Health Promotion/Mental Health Services/School Nurses, Nutrition Education, Safe and Drug Free Schools Program, 21st Century Community Learning Centers/After-school programs, Family Resource Centers, Young Parents Program, and Education of Homeless Children and Youth. Ms. Russell-Tucker is past president of the Connecticut Dietetic Association and of the CACFP National Professional Association. She is also an adjunct faculty member at a local college where she teaches business management courses in the program for nontraditional students. She received her M.S. in management from Albertus Magnus College–New Dimensions in New Haven, Connecticut, and is a registered dietitian.

VIRGINIA A. STALLINGS, M.D., is the Jean A. Cortner Endowed Chair in Pediatric Gastroenterology, Director of the Nutrition Center, and Director of the Office of Faculty Development at the Children's Hospital of Philadelphia Research Institute. Dr. Stallings is also Professor of Pediatrics at the University of Pennsylvania School of Medicine. Her research interests include pediatric nutrition, evaluation of dietary intake and energy expenditure, and nutrition-related chronic disease. Dr. Stallings recently served as chair of the IOM Committee on Nutrition Standards for National School Lunch and Breakfast Programs. She has previously served on the Committee on Nutrition Standards for Foods in Schools (chair), the Committee on Nutrition Services for Medicare Beneficiaries (chair), the Committee on the Scientific Basis for Dietary Risk Eligibility Criteria for WIC Programs (chair), and the Committee to Review the WIC Food Packages (member). She is a former member of the Food and Nutrition Board. Dr. Stallings earned a B.S. degree in nutrition and foods from Auburn University, an M.S. degree in human nutrition and biochemistry from Cornell University, and an M.D. from the School of Medicine of the University of Alabama in Birmingham. She completed a pediatric residency at the University of Virginia and a nutrition fellowship at the Hospital for Sick Children, Toronto, Ontario. Dr. Stallings is board certified in pediatrics and clinical nutrition. She has been an IOM member since 2005 and recently received the Foman Nutrition Award from the American Academy of Pediatrics.

KATHERINE L. TUCKER, Ph.D., is Professor and Chair, Department of Health Sciences, at Northeastern University. Previously she was Senior Scientist and Director of the Dietary Assessment and Epidemiology Research Program at the USDA Human Nutrition Research Center on Aging at Tufts University, and Professor and Director of the Nutritional Epidemiology Program for the Gerald J. and Dorothy R. Friedman School of Nutrition Science and Policy at Tufts University, where she holds an adjunct appointment. Her research interests include diet and health, nutrition in older adults, dietary methodology, nutritional status of high-risk populations, and nutritional epidemiology. She previously served on the IOM Committee on the Implications of Dioxin in the Food Supply. Dr. Tucker is an Associate Editor for the *Journal of Nutrition* and is currently the incoming chair of the Nutritional Sciences Council of the American Society for Nutrition. In addition, she is a member of the American Society for Bone and Mineral Research and the Gerontological Society of America. Dr. Tucker received her B.Sc. in nutritional sciences from the University of Connecticut and her Ph.D. in nutrition sciences from Cornell University.

C

Workshop Agenda: February 2010

Improving CACFP Through Research,
Outreach, and Implementation:
A Workshop for the Committee to Review
Child and Adult Care Food Program Meal Requirements

The National Academy of Sciences
2100 C Street, NW
Washington, DC
Lecture Room

February 23, 2010

8:00–9:00 am   Registration

INTRODUCTION

9:00   Welcome
                 *Suzanne Murphy, Ph.D., R.D., Chair, Committee to
                 Review Child and Adult Care Food Programs*

SESSION 1: CACFP RESEARCH

9:10   Promoting Healthy Eating and Physical Activity in CACFP
                 Lorrene Ritchie, Ph.D., University of California, Berkeley

9:30   Environmental Influences on Eating Behavior of Children
                Marlene Schwartz, Ph.D., Yale University

9:50   Q&A

10:00   BREAK

SESSION 2: OUTREACH—VOICES FROM THE PROGRAMS

10:30   Adult Day Care Program Issues
                Michael S. Young DiGeronimo R.D., Madison
                  Adult Day Health Care Center, Arlington
                  County Department of Human Services, VA

                Donna Cross, The Support Center, Montgomery
                  County, MD

10:50   Child Care Program Issues
                Everludis Lopez R.D., Head Start, Fairfax, VA

                Tanya Matthews, Latin American Community Center,
                  Wilmington, DE

11:10   Q&A

SESSION 3: PROGRESS IN PROGRAM IMPLEMENTATION

11:30   Best Practices for Obesity Prevention and Health
                  Promotion
                Debbie Chang, M.P.H., Nemours, Delaware

11:50   Healthy Meal Patterns in CACFP: New York State's
                  Perspective
                Lynn Ouderkerk, M.A., R.D., Center for Community
                  Health, New York State Department of Health

12:10 pm   Q&A

12:30   Potential Impact of Type of Retail Outlets on CACFP
                  Food Costs
                Ephraim Leibtag, Ph.D., Economic Research Service,
                  U.S. Department of Agriculture, Washington, D.C.

12:50   Q&A

1:00   Adjourn

Appendixes D through M are not printed in this book but can be found on the CD at the back of the book or online at http://www.nap.edu.

Index

E

N